Multiple
Sclerosis

and Having a Baby

Multiple Sclerosis
and Having a Baby

**Everything You Need to Know
about Conception, Pregnancy,
and Parenthood**

JUDY GRAHAM

Healing Arts Press
Rochester, Vermont

Healing Arts Press
One Park Street
Rochester, Vermont 05767
www.InnerTraditions.com

Healing Arts Press is a division of Inner Traditions International

Note to the reader: This book is intended as an informational guide. The remedies, approaches, and techniques described herein are meant to supplement, and not to be a substitute for, professional medical care or treatment. They should not be used to treat a serious ailment without prior consultation with a qualified health care professional.

LIBRARY OF CONGRESS CATALOGING-IN-PUBLICATION DATA

Graham, Judy.
    Multiple sclerosis and having a baby : everything you need to know about conception, pregnancy, and parenthood / Judy Graham.
    p. cm.
    ISBN 0-89281-788-7 (alk. paper)
    1. Pregnancy in physically handicapped women.   2. Pregnant women—Diseases—Complications.   3. Multiple sclerosis—Complications.   I. Title.
RG580.P48G73   1999
618.3—dc21   99-18416
                                                                              CIP

Printed and bound in Canada

10 9 8 7 6 5 4 3 2 1

Text design and layout by Jenna Dixon
This book was typeset in Century Schoolbook with Eras as the display typeface

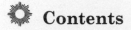 **Contents**

✳ Acknowledgments

I wish to thank the many people who generously gave their time to tell of their own experiences and passed on their tips and wisdom. For the sake of confidentiality, their names have been changed except where credited. Particular thanks to Cathy from Long Island, New York; Lauri from Los Angeles, California; Sue and daughter Steph from Seattle, Washington; Danny from Chicago, Illinois; Emily from Montreal, Canada; Jeanne from Warsaw, Indiana; Leona from Danbury, Connecticut; Maria from Columbus, Ohio; Maribeth from Ogden, Utah; Marcy from Charleston, South Carolina; Mellanie from Phoenix, Arizona; Tracey from Burlington, Vermont; Gordon from Hartsdale, New York; Julie from San Antonio, Texas; Jon from Atlanta, Georgia; Lyndsy from Madison, Wisconsin; Sandra from Newburyport, Massachusetts; Robin from Newbury, Massachusetts; Lilian from Lexington, Kentucky; Naomi from Toronto, Canada; Elena from Pittsburgh, Pennsylvania; Sarah from Annapolis, Maryland; and John Pageler from Pinellas Park, Florida. Thanks also to Jo O'Farrell, Janet Bradshaw, Beverley James, Jacquie Kent, Michele Wates, Rachel Shrimpton, Mark Shrimpton, Gillian Beck, Elizabeth Brice, Michelle Leon, Jayne Harrison, Gill Heath, David Millett, Paul Powell, Alex Cowan, Diana McGovern, Yvette McAngus, Professor Michael Barnes, and Dr. Sally Field.

I have drawn from published work written by doctors who are experts in this field, particularly Dr. Kathy Birk, Dr. Richard Rudick, and Dr. Cassandra Henderson. I wish to thank the National Multiple Sclerosis Society for their information and knowledge and all the many MS organizations on the World Wide Web who helped me find the cases quoted in this book. Acknowledgments to the researchers on Complementary Therapies in MS, particularly Jo Barnes from Exeter University, England. My partner, Samuel Long, was a great help in checking through the manuscript and making wise, perceptive, and astute suggestions. Last, special thanks to my fourteen-year-old son, Pascal, who cooked and served up many meals while I worked.

✳ Introduction

Will my symptoms get worse if I have a baby? And how will I be able to look after my child? These are the key questions asked by women with multiple sclerosis. The best place to find the answers is from other people, and that's exactly the purpose of this book—to provide answers from the experiences of other people with MS. Based on the stories of dozens of parents with MS, this book tells what it's like being a mother or father with MS, covering every aspect of the disease, pregnancy, and parenthood. Besides individual stories, it also gives all the latest scientific facts on this subject, both positive and negative. With *all* the facts both good and bad— you can be fully prepared for whatever decision you make.

As you will see, the medical authorities do not totally agree with one another. Even so, the general conclusion is good news: Women with MS who have children are no worse off in the long run than those who do not.

Being a parent with MS is not easy. Sometimes it's heartbreakingly difficult. Even though the book has some sad stories, it also has many happy ones. No matter what happened to them, nearly everyone is glad they had children.

I have to admit to a bias in writing this book. As a mother with MS, I wholeheartedly support having children. A child makes your life so much fuller, richer, and more joyful. A child gives a dimension to life that you otherwise wouldn't experience. A child makes you think of someone else first; a child makes you plan for the future.

My Own Story

I gave birth to Pascal in 1985, when I was thirty-eight years old and had had MS for at least twelve years. He was born at home, totally naturally. The labor lasted just over three hours and was easy. I started breast-feeding immediately and carried on for more than three years. Pascal is now fourteen. Even though I say so myself, he is tall, dark, handsome, charming, witty, and smart. He also makes a mean BLT sandwich. As you can tell, I love my son a lot. I haven't been the kind of mother who could run along beaches or join him in bike rides. I haven't baked cakes or sewn drapes. I spend much of my life sitting down. But does that make me less of a mother? I don't think so, and neither does he.

Ten Good Reasons to Have a Child

🖋 *"Don't let MS stop you from having children. They are the greatest gift from God, and they make your life better than you ever dreamed!"*

🖋 *"Children give you hugs and kisses. It's wonderful."*

🖋 *"If I didn't have children, I would probably lie in bed all day feeling sorry for myself and then my MS would get worse. I don't have time to think of how I'm feeling because I'm too busy being a mom."*

🖋 *"It's such a joy to see how they develop. I wouldn't be without my boys for the world, even though my MS has gotten worse."*

🖋 *"My son has taught me so much. God gives you children so that you can learn from them and learn about yourself. I would have put up with anything to have this child, no matter how bad the exacerbation."*

🖋 *"I couldn't bear not having children. I would rather look back and think it's been hard than never to have done it at all."*

🖋 *"Hang on and enjoy the ride—talk about a roller-coaster ride."*

🖋 *"MS has taken away so much from my life, but I'm not having motherhood taken away from me. I can have a baby, and I know I can be a good mother."*

🖋 *"Having a child gives some purpose to life. No matter how bad your day may be, you've got this child who's dependent on you and whose love is number one."*

🖋 *"When I look at the kids, I can see what I have to be happy about rather than letting the disease eat me alive and feeling sorry for myself. Children give you a reason to live. They give you an energy to go on that you wouldn't have if you were by yourself. You don't dwell on your problems because you have someone depending on you and it's your job to take care of them."*

- Will pregnancy make my MS worse, in either the short or the long term?

- Will I pass on MS to my children?

- Do I need any special prenatal care because I have MS?

- Will MS affect my labor or delivery?

- What pain relief is safe for me during labor?

- What effect does an abortion have on MS?

- Can I lessen my risk of having a relapse after the baby is born?

- Should I breast-feed?

- What drugs are safe to take during pregnancy and while breast-feeding?

- Will MS affect my ability to look after my baby?

TOP TEN TIPS

- Plan to get help once the baby is born. You may not think you need it now, but you may come to need it later.

- Think about who you can rely on for help. Ask them in advance.

- Don't be afraid to ask for help.

- Talk things through with your husband or partner. He may have to do more than he bargained for.

- Involve your family. You'll need everyone's support.

- Don't try to do it all, or you'll end up exhausted.

- Be realistic about the future. Plan for the worst, and hope for the best.

- Make decisions about your lifestyle that make things easier for you, not harder.

- Try to meet other mothers with MS. Role models help.

- Don't let MS rule your life.

COMMON FEARS OF PREGNANT WOMEN WITH MS

- Falling while they're pregnant
- Dropping the baby after delivery
- Not being a "normal" mother
- Passing on MS to their babies
- Labor bringing on an MS attack

1 ☼ Will I Get Worse If I Have a Baby?

First the good news . . . The good news is that you will probably be healthier during *pregnancy* than at any other time. Relapses are less likely during pregnancy. This is because the hormones in a woman's body during pregnancy seem to have a good effect on the immune system.

Then the bad news . . . The bad news is that you run a high risk of having a relapse in the first six months after giving birth. The first three months are the riskiest. Up to 70 percent of women with MS have some sort of relapse in the first three months after having a baby.[1]

But there is more good news . . . Relapses in the first six months following childbirth usually make no difference to long-term disability.

Multiple sclerosis is most likely to be diagnosed just at the time when young adults are thinking of starting a family, facing them with a dilemma about whether or not to become parents. Not so long ago, neurologists advised women with MS against getting pregnant. They thought that having a baby made MS worse and that women with MS would not be able to look after a baby properly. But today doctors are much more likely to say, "Go ahead and have one"—as long as you have social support. Dr. Cassandra Henderson, the Associate Director of Obstetrics and Perinatology at Jack D. Weiler Hospital, says that what concerns her most is not a woman's disorder, but her social situation.

One reason for this change of tune is research. Many new studies have found that women with MS are usually very well during pregnancy. And although there is an increased risk of relapse in the first six months after giving birth, having a baby does not generally alter the course of MS, nor does it make it worse in the long run. With support, mothers and fathers with MS can look after their babies perfectly well.

The introduction of new medications for MS has also changed the picture and made it more positive. But the new treatments affect the timing of having a baby. Some doctors think it is sensible to have a baby before starting drug treatment, since you can't take the drugs while you're pregnant, trying to become pregnant, or nursing.

Pregnancy

Most women with MS feel better than ever during pregnancy. Relapses are fewer and women enjoy good health. MS often stabilizes during pregnancy and sometimes improves. Relapses can happen during pregnancy, but they tend to be fewer than at other times. In one study[2] it was found that disease activity declined during the second half of pregnancy.

🖋 *"I was absolutely wonderful during the pregnancy. I wish they could find out why pregnancy makes women feel so well and bottle it!"*

🖋 *"I didn't have any major symptoms. I was able to walk normally and never thought about whether it would get worse."*

🖋 *"Pregnancy had no visible effects on my MS one way or the other."*

☛ *"When I was pregnant I was the healthiest I have ever been. Even with my big tummy, I could walk five blocks. I wasn't able to do that before, and I haven't been able to do it since."*

Immune Suppression during Pregnancy

One reason for the lower rate of relapse during pregnancy is that immune suppression occurs at this time.[3] MS is considered to be an auto-immune disease in which the immune system mistakenly attacks itself, so although the exact mechanisms of action are unclear, immune suppression results in fewer symptoms. A complicated network of interactions among the immune, hormonal, and nervous systems probably explains the favorable effects of pregnancy. During pregnancy there are a number of substances present in a woman's body, such as alpha-fetoprotein, that may have a good effect on the immune system. Estrogen and progesterone, both of which reach high levels, have strong modulating effects on the immune system too.

John N. Whitaker, M.D., a neurologist at the University of Alabama in Birmingham, Alabama, suggests the following mechanism:

> Several alterations in immunologic status occur during pregnancy, among them an apparent shift from a predominance of type 1, or proinflammatory, helper T cells, to type 2, or anti-inflammatory helper cells, with a reversal after pregnancy. . . . Proinflammatory helper T cells appear to have an important role in the pathogenesis of multiple sclerosis. The influence of anti-inflammatory helper cells in the mother during the last trimester of pregnancy may lead to suppression of disease, which then escapes control when the shift from anti-inflammatory to

Pregnancy has a favorable effect on the course of multiple sclerosis on both a long-term and short-term basis.[4]

The conditions of most women with MS stabilize or improve during pregnancy. . . . exacerbation rates are reduced to about half that expected in non-pregnant patients with MS.[5]

Relapses occurring during pregnancy were generally mild or moderate and left no or minimal residual disability.[6]

Despite early reports to the contrary, pregnancy is now generally considered to provide a stabilizing effect on the clinical course of MS.[7]

Pregnancy does not appear to be a period of greater risk for exacerbations, but, on the contrary, it seems to act, on the whole, as a protective event. These data allow physicians to provide reassuring counselling to women.[8]

proinflammatory helper T cells occurs during the postpartum period.[9]

Some scientists say it makes sense to isolate the protective factors during pregnancy and develop them for use as a treatment. The animal model for MS, experimental allergic encephalomyelitis, has been treated with limited success with alpha-fetoprotein. A vaccine against rheumatoid arthritis that re-creates some of the conditions of pregnancy is currently under development.

Attacks during Pregnancy

Even though women are often better during pregnancy than at other times, relapses can happen. One study of 125 patients found that although relapses were significantly reduced during pregnancy, they still occurred and were occasionally severe.[10]

🖋 *"When I was about three or four months pregnant with my first daughter I was twenty years old. I developed a cold, wet, burning sensation all down my left leg and into my foot. The doctor thought it could be a pinched nerve, or a blood clot, or whatever, but he couldn't really do any testing. It was only after the baby was born that I realized it was an MS attack."*

🖋 *"Around eleven or twelve weeks into the pregnancy I started having bladder problems. I couldn't pee. I would sit for twenty minutes and push with all my might and run water and everything, but I couldn't go."*

The Risk of Relapse after Having a Baby

There is no hiding the fact that there is an increased risk of relapse in the first six months after having a baby. You stand roughly a fifty-fifty chance of having an attack at this time. Which means you also stand a fifty-fifty chance of *not* having a relapse.

Relapse means a recurrence of MS signs and symptoms the patient had before or the onset of new ones. The official length of time a relapse lasts is more than 24 hours and less than two months. Anything less might be called an "episode."

Anything longer is probably not a relapse but a symptom which is part of chronic-progressive MS. The severity can range from mild to terrible. A relapse can include some or all of the following symptoms: gait disturbance, sensory loss, shaky movements, staggering walk, fatigue, paralysis of any limb, optic neuritis, increased weakness, bowel and bladder problems, or depression.

Relapses in the six months after childbirth can also be more severe than usual. This may be because of the changes in hormone levels at this time. The first six months after childbirth is generally considered to be one of the three most risky times for women with MS. (The others are puberty and menopause.) If you have been prone to exacerbations in the course of your MS, you are more likely to have one in the six months after the baby is born. The exacerbations are rarely permanent, however. After this period, relapses tend to go back to their prepregnancy level and the relapses that occur in the six months after having a baby tend not to make any difference to long-term disability.

Women with MS have a wide range of experiences following the births of their babies. Some noticeably worsen during the first year; others stay stable, while others may have relapses from which they partially recover.

🐾 *"When she was six months old, my walking started to go downhill. And from eighteen months, I was in a wheelchair all the time."*

🐾 *"I got as tired as any woman would normally get with a new baby. MS didn't really affect me. It was just there, that's all."*

What the Medical Literature Says about Relapses in the Six Months after Having a Baby

As compared with the year before conception, there was a decrease of about 70 percent in the rate of relapse during the third trimester of pregnancy, followed by an increase of about 70 percent over the prepregnancy rate in the first three months postpartum.[11]

Fifty-three percent of full-term pregnancies were followed by a relapse.[12]

The study suggested that the risk of clinical relapse after delivery may be higher than has been reported previously. Six of eight women (75 percent) experienced a flare-up in their MS postpartum. This was 10 times the rate observed in the same women during gestation.[13]

Between 20 percent and 40 percent of patients with MS will experience a clinical relapse or worsening of the disease during the three months after delivery.[14]

During the first 3 months following delivery there was a sharp increase of relapse rate. . . . Relapses tended to be more severe.[15]

The greatest risk of MS exacerbation occurred in the first three months after childbirth; 68 percent of postpartum exacerbations occurred during this period. The exacerbation rate appeared to stabilize beyond the six months after childbirth.[16]

The mean disability score worsened in this population of patients with MS from 2.4 late in pregnancy to 2.8 at 6 weeks postpartum and to 3.4 at 6 months postpartum.[17]

🪶 *"MS has just progressed in the usual way. Having two children hasn't made much difference."*

🪶 *"I was fine until the baby was nine months old, and I thought I'd gotten away with it. And then—bam!—I couldn't walk."*

🪶 *"Within hours of the birth I developed bladder incontinence."*

🪶 *"You can't live your life always thinking, what if? No one knows what's around the corner anyway. You can't let MS rule your life."*

The worst case scenario for a new mother with MS would be to have an attack and never fully recover. Others have attacks but get over them. The lucky ones—and there are many of them — sail through their child's first year without any flare-up of MS at all. Although it is unusual, there are some women who regret having had a child because their MS deteriorated afterward.

While there is no way of knowing what will happen in any particular case, the following stories illustrate the wide range of what can happen in the months after a baby is born.

"It's the Worst I've Ever Been" ☼ Liz's Story

"I had a very bad relapse after my first son was born. It happened about six weeks after the birth. It's the worst I've ever been. I couldn't walk at all and had a lot of pain down my side. It was really horrible pain. They wanted to put me on steroids, but I didn't want to take them. I think the relapse was undoubtedly to do with having the baby. But I was really mad because I didn't think things through before the baby was born. I just assumed I'd be able to manage, looking after the baby and doing the housework. But I couldn't.

"With the second one, I made sure I had plenty of help and I stayed in bed a lot and got plenty of rest. That time I was perfectly OK and didn't have a relapse. With hindsight, I should have done the same for the first one."

"Nothing Happened at All" ☼ Lilian's Story

"I have very happy memories of my son's first year. I never had a relapse, and my walking was good enough to go for lovely, long, springtime walks with him. I had had mild MS attacks when I was first diagnosed—arms, hands, or feet going numb or pins and needles—but during those first twelve months nothing happened at all. I was just like any other mother. Since then, my MS has deteriorated, but just slowly over the years and without any relapses. Having a baby made no difference to my MS, and I can't imagine life without him."

"If I'd Known What Was Going to Happen, I Definitely Would Not Have Had a Baby" ☼ Jennifer's Story

"I definitely got worse after having my baby. It happened five weeks after the birth. My legs just said, 'That's it—I've had enough!' The doctor never told me anything about any risk, and it never crossed my mind that I might get worse since I'd had eight years of remission. But with hindsight, if I'd known what was going to happen, I definitely would not have had a baby.

"Before I had my son I was able to do a very energetic job out on the farm. I rode horses every morning at five. But now I'm so bad all I can do is my husband's book work. I'm very weak on my legs and use a cane plus hold on to walls. I do sometimes think I wouldn't be like this if I hadn't had a child. If a woman with MS came to me asking for my advice, I'd tell her my story and tell her that if I'd known what was going to happen, I wouldn't have gone ahead and had a child, even though I love him to bits."

How to Reduce the Risk of a Relapse

A new mother is on call twenty-four hours a day, with interrupted nights and lack of sleep. Moreover, once the baby is born, the hormonal and other factors that modulated the immune system return to their prepregnancy state. While the results of studies on the causes of relapse are not clear-cut, common sense suggests that physical and emotional strain are front-runners as triggers for a relapse.

TIPS TO REDUCE THE CHANCE OF HAVING A RELAPSE

- Get enough rest.
- Get undisturbed sleep.
- Don't overdo things.
- Get treatment for anemia.
- Minimize stress.
- Avoid infection.
- Avoid getting too hot.

Does Having a Baby Make MS Worse in the Long Run?

The most recent study to research this, carried out in Birmingham, Alabama, found: "There was no effect on the overall rate of disease progression during the 33-month study period, which included the year before pregnancy, the pregnancy itself, and the year after delivery."[21]

The general view is that having a baby does not alter the overall course of MS, including long-term disability, but some researchers urge caution. In some cases, severe relapses in the first six months after childbirth can have lasting effects. What type of MS you have can make a difference. The medical studies have tended to focus on the 80 to 90 percent of women with the relapsing/remitting type of MS. The 10 to 20 percent of women with the progressive form, who suffer the greatest permanent disability, may do worse when they have babies.[22] The positive figures about long-term outcome may also be influenced by the fact that younger and less disabled women with a better MS prognosis are more likely to have children than those who are older, more disabled, and who have a poorer prognosis.

One three-year study reached this conclusion.

Despite papers showing no effect of pregnancy on disability in large groups of women, some women do deteriorate post partum and do not recover. It may be that these are the progressive from onset patients, and they should be investigated separately before stating that there are no long-term effects of pregnancy on MS.[23]

Types of MS and Having a Baby

Dr. Cassandra Henderson says,

I would make *very* sure you understand the course your MS might follow both during and immediately after pregnancy. You should understand that while MS is an unpredictable disease, the severity and duration of your previous exacerbations are the best clues to predicting your future illness.

What happens to you when you have a baby depends to some extent on the type of MS you have. It is sometimes not fully explained to women that there is not just one kind of MS. There are two distinct types:

- **Relapsing/Remitting MS:** This type is characterized by attacks that come and then go away again. In the beginning, you go back to being symptom-free after an attack. But as time goes on, or if attacks are severe, there is usually some residual damage.

- **Progressive MS:** This is the type where there are no distinct relapses or remissions. Instead, the disease steadily progresses. You can also develop secondary progressive MS. Many people start by having the relapsing/remitting kind of MS, then after a certain period of time the disease becomes secondary progressive—relapses stop, but disease progression continues.

At the positive end of the spectrum is benign MS. Attacks are mild and infrequent, leaving virtually no disabling symptoms. Life span and lifestyle can be virtually normal. At the other end of the spectrum, MS can sometimes progress very rapidly with severe symptoms. In this small percentage of cases, life expectancy is dramatically shortened, and the person is significantly disabled. Between these two extremes lie most cases of MS. There is no guarantee that your course will stay the same throughout your life. It can sometimes happen that mild MS becomes more severe, perhaps after some stressful life event. Even though MS is said to be an unpredictable disease, the severity of relapses, how often they happen, and the damage they leave behind can predict to some extent what will happen in the course of the disease in each case.

Women with mild MS and less disability are more likely to have a baby and to get the full go-ahead from their doctors. Women with more severe MS and a greater degree of disability are more likely to give their doctors concern. Dr. Henderson cautions,

> If you are a woman with a permanent or severe disability, I would carefully and fully discuss the social situation. It is key on two counts. One: the course of the pregnancy and the postpartum situation can be somewhat more complex as a result of disability. The possibility of an exacerbation after delivery is increased, although, on the whole, an exacerbation is not any more permanent for a woman with more disability than for a woman with mild MS. Two: after the child is born, adequate support is more likely to be required than in the case of an asymptomatic woman.

What If You Do Have a Relapse?

The first step is to get help so that other people can look after the baby and do the cooking, the shopping, and all the household chores. If possible, you should not be separated from your baby. The priority for the baby is that you are physically *there*. Your presence is more important than anything you actually do.

If you have a relapse bad enough to send you to the hospital, talk it through with your doctor to see whether you can have treatment at home instead. If not, try to arrange for someone to bring your baby to the hospital as often as possible. Even though it will be distressing for the baby—and you —to be parted from each other, it is better for the baby to see his or her mother in the hospital than to not see her at all.

If you do have a bad relapse shortly after having a baby, you may feel you made a mistake in having a child. This is a common feeling, but almost always short-lived. The temporary feelings of regret and of having made a mistake disappear when the relapse subsides and you experience the joy of your child once again.

Going Back to Work

Women in full-time employment may be given only six to eight weeks of maternity leave. This may cause problems for women with MS, since the time after childbirth is a period of high risk for a relapse. Work is one of the factors that should be fully discussed before having a baby. If you have not told your employer that you have MS, it can cause additional stress.

Some women manage to succeed in the juggling act of being a working mother with MS by following a regime that maximizes their health and well-being. The following comes from a physician who herself has MS.

"Was Giving Life to Her Worth Feeling So Bad?" ☼ Jeanne's Story

"I remember literally crawling down the hall to my daughter's room to take care of her. I really wondered if I had made the right decision. Was giving life to her worth feeling so bad that I wanted to die? I felt like I'd been hit by a truck, had the flu, and had a horrible hangover all the time.

"Now, thanks to sticking to a low-fat diet, my MS is mild and I am fine. My memories of that horrible time have now faded. If I could choose again whether to have that child or not I would say a resounding *yes!* My kids give my life meaning, and I believe I do better with this disease because of them.

I wouldn't have missed motherhood for the world. My kids were the big reason I couldn't consider suicide when I was so sick and depressed back in 1987. I knew it was better for them to have a sick, disabled mother than one who took the easy way out by killing herself."

Can Having a Baby Trigger MS?

🖋 *"My baby has just turned a year old. I'm still not diagnosed with MS, but I suspect I have it. I've been noticing weird things bit by bit, and I now have quite a few symptoms."*

For the first half of this century, it was believed that having a baby could trigger MS—that there was a definite cause and effect relationship. Now, scientists aren't sure. Some say there is a higher risk of MS onset at this time; others say there isn't. Maybe it's just coincidence—a first attack of MS usually happens during childbearing years.

"It Seemed Like the World Was Coming to an End" ☼ Julie's Story

"When Heather was about five weeks old, things started to happen. My left eye had this pain and what seemed like a film over it. This lasted for a month. I put it off and put it off and finally couldn't stand the pain anymore and made an appointment to see an opthalmologist, thinking I had an eye infection or something.

"He looked into my eyes and started asking me questions. Then he made an appointment for me to see an optic neurologist. From there things went downhill. By the time I got to see the neurologist, I was barely walking and then was hospitalized after that. My mom and dad drove from Indiana to

Virginia to see me and find out what was going on. It was very scary. For the next year things were touch and go, mostly with my eyes. A lot of optic neuritis and tingles and numbness, but nothing major, although at the time it seemed like the world was coming to an end."

Sometimes it can look like having a baby has triggered MS. But in fact a woman may have had symptoms years before. Her doctor may have had suspicions of MS, but may have waited to tell her until after the birth of a baby. This was the case with Emily, a Canadian woman.

"My Legs Wouldn't Do What I Wanted Them to Do" ☼ Emily's Story

"I was diagnosed with MS a little over a month ago. I'm twenty-five and the mother of two. I presented symptoms of MS after the birth of my son a little more than three years ago: numbness, loss of vision. My doctor had me have tests, but nothing was conclusive. For the next few years I had the same symptoms, only worse, but I dismissed it.

"I got pregnant again and delivered a healthy baby girl in February 1998. About three weeks after the delivery, I would get dizzy for no reason. I could be sitting or standing. Many times I wouldn't be able to see out of one eye; sometimes both eyes would be impaired. I started to fall, almost as if my legs wouldn't do what I wanted them to do. My hands would get stiff. It seemed like everything was getting stiff. I was also dropping things, numb, and extremely tired. Everything was getting to be very difficult (an understatement!).

"I was also trying to hide the symptoms from my husband. I tried putting all this down to the stress of a new baby on top of moving just two weeks after she was born. It finally came

What the Medical Literature Says about Pregnancy or Childbirth Triggering MS

In the first four decades of this century, several studies have demonstrated that 10–20 percent of women with MS had onset after pregnancy or childbirth, and this finding led to the conclusion that pregnancy or childbirth could trigger MS. . . . There are studies confirming the earlier findings.[24]

In agreement with others, our data show that the risk of onset and deterioration of MS is particularly high shortly after childbirth. This phenomenon is still poorly understood.[25]

to a head when I was unable to get my words out and my speech was slurred. When I could no longer hide things, I went to the doctor. The diagnosis of MS was made after an MRI scan, which clearly showed MS plaques."

Can Having a Baby Offer Protection?

There is no doubt that in the first six months after a baby is born, there is a high risk of relapse. However, in the long term, women with MS who have had a child can do better than those who do not have children. A variety of documented studies on the subject have reached these conclusions:

- Mothers are at lower risk of getting MS than childless women.[26]
- Childless women with MS have a higher relapse rate than MS women who have had children.[27]

- There is a significantly decreased risk of a progressive course of the disease in women who got pregnant after MS was diagnosed, this protection against deterioration lasting for several years.[28]

- Patients who had at least one pregnancy after onset of MS were wheelchair dependent after 18.6 years versus 12.5 years for other women.[29]

- Women with pregnancies during MS tended to have a more benign prognosis. . . . Patients with a younger age at onset, in general, had a better prognosis than late-onset patients, and younger patients were more likely to become pregnant during the disease.[30]

- MS mothers with onset during pregnancy had significantly less disability than the other groups.[31]

Timing of Pregnancy

One group of researchers compared women with MS who had no children with mothers whose diagnosis of MS was made before pregnancy, during pregnancy, and after pregnancy. The group that did the best were those who were diagnosed *during* pregnancy. A group of German researchers[32] found that women who had had a baby *after* the diagnosis of MS tended to be less disabled than women who had had a baby *before* the diagnosis of MS. They think, however, that the difference in disability has more to do with the woman's age at MS onset, rather than with her age at giving birth. Patients who became pregnant only *after* a diagnosis of MS were younger (the mean age at onset was 22.5 years) whereas patients who had become pregnant *before* diagnosis were older (the mean age at onset was 34.5 years).

- MS usually develops between the ages of twenty and forty.

- MS is nearly twice as common in women as in men.

- Women tend to have a more benign disease course and, on average, a better outcome.[33]

- The average time lapse between MS diagnosis and becoming pregnant is three and a half years.

- There is no difference in prognosis between women who have never had children and men.

- Women with MS are more likely to be childless and less likely to be married.

- In a Swedish study, of 153 women with MS, 74 had never had children. In a normal population, for women of childbearing age, that figure would be 50.

- In the same study, only 94 women were married. In a normal population, the expected figure would be 104.

2 ❋ Can You Pass MS on to Your Child?

Often, women contemplating having children are more concerned about the possible risks to their children than about
the risks to themselves. Some feel a real sense of fear that
their children could develop MS later on; others never give it
a second thought.

🐾 *"Four of my cousins have MS. One got much worse after
having a baby and has now died. So we were worried
about any genetic connection. We went to see a neurologist
who's doing research into familial links, and he said: 'Go
away and get a baby under your belt.'"*

🐾 *"I am terrified my boy will get MS. It really haunts me."*

🐾 *"I've never worried about a genetic connection. I haven't
let it bother me."*

🐾 *"We talked to a doctor about whether MS is hereditary.
The doctor told us it was a higher risk among families, but
not hereditary. So we decided to go ahead and have the
baby."*

Genetic Susceptibility

MS is not hereditary in the same way as, say, hemophilia,
which is passed on unfailingly. But there is a familial link.
This means that where there is MS already in the family,
there could be a genetic susceptibility. It has been calculated
that children born to a parent with MS have a 3 to 5 percent

lifetime risk of MS, compared with a 0.1 percent risk for the general population. They also have a 95 to 97 percent chance of *not* getting MS. If you have a relative affected by MS, it is up to seven times more likely than normal for the general population that MS will affect you. There are some families that have clusters of MS, with the condition appearing in several members over two or more generations. These clusters are unusual and slightly distort the overall figures.

Females seem to be more at risk than males. The risk to a child is greater when the mother rather than the father is affected. The highest risk transfers from mothers to daughters. The risk for a daughter of a woman with MS is 4.96 percent (fifty times greater than the general population) until about the age of twenty-eight, when it drops to 2.5 percent. By the age of thirty-three, the risk is down to 1.5 percent and falls as low as 0.5 percent by the age of forty-three. The risk for an identical twin being affected is 25.9 percent. This is markedly higher than the rate for nonidentical twins, who do not share the same genetic material—2.3 percent.

The largest and most systematic study ever conducted on the risk of relatives getting MS took place in British Columbia, Canada.[1] Researchers found that 20 percent of patients with MS had at least one relative with MS, possible MS, or optic neuritis. Some people who get MS have particular gene markers called histocompatability complex antigens (HLAs). A few HLA types are commonly seen in MS. These tissue types are also widespread in healthy people, and for this reason they are not a sufficient predictor of MS on their own. About 45 percent of people with MS have the particular HLAs associated with MS, but so do 25 percent of the general population.

What the Medical Literature Says about the Genetic Risk of MS

Family studies have clearly shown that relatives of patients are at a substantially increased risk for developing the disease compared with the general population. In general, children and siblings of MS patients have a risk to develop the disease that is 30 to 50 times greater than of the general population.[2]*

---

*The study cited was done in British Columbia, Canada—a high risk area for MS. The data are relevant only to other areas of high risk.

3 ✸ Deciding Whether to Have a Baby

🖉 *"There are a lot of women out there who are torn between having children and not having children."*

🖉 *"We started talking about having a baby like any other couple. MS was never a great factor. The whole thing is an unknown anyway."*

The decision whether to have a baby is a very personal one. Each woman with MS must weigh a number of issues: how much she wants a child, her own health, the possibility of getting worse, whether she can look after her child herself or must get help. Other factors are her partner's attitude, the financial impact on the family, and how a baby would affect her career. Dr. Cassandra Henderson says her final advice on the subject is a question. "Why do you and your partner want a child? In the last analysis, the joy of raising a child often overcomes many of the problems associated with MS and child-rearing."

Doctors Kathy Birk and Richard Rudick, who have conducted extensive research on MS and childbearing, say,

> The decision to become a parent should rest primarily on the desire to have a family. But the current degree of physical impairment and support available from the father, friends, and relatives are important considerations. . . . The unpredictable and potentially disabling nature of the disease makes careful counseling and judicious treatment critical.

Dr. Birk is a clinical instructor of obstetrics and gynecology at the University of Rochester School of Medicine. Dr. Rudick directs the Mellen Center for Multiple Sclerosis Treatment and Research in Cleveland.

Experts at the International Federation of Multiple Sclerosis Societies warn that

> It is very important to remember that child-rearing is a long-term commitment and couples must think about the impact of MS over the eighteen years or so during which they will be actively involved in raising a child, and not concentrate just on pregnancy and the newborn period.

One recent study on MS and childbearing concluded that, "Decisions against childbearing that relate to MS can usually be attributed to physical disability that precludes child care, or to recommendations from physicians that are based on opinion and attitudes prevalent in the first half of the century."[1] Doctors Birk and Rudick sum up those outdated attitudes in one of their articles.

> Virtually all published case reports and reviews before 1949 concluded that pregnancy adversely affected MS. Some authors warned against pregnancy because of possible transmission of disease to the infant; others raised concerns about inadequate mothering. This led physicians as late as 1950 to routinely recommend that patients with MS avoid pregnancy and that pregnant patients with MS electively terminate their pregnancies and consider sterilization.[2]*

Wise Up and Plan Carefully

Some doctors may tell you to go away and forget you have MS altogether. It is probably wiser to take it into account if

---

*"Pregnancy" in this context means the nine months of gestation plus the three months after the baby is born.

you do plan to have a baby because you will almost certainly need to make practical, financial, psychological, and emotional adjustments.

"It Would Have Been Better If He'd Said: 'Go Away and Adapt Your Life'" ☼ Michele's Story

"When I was first diagnosed with MS, the neurologist said to me, 'This is an incurable disease. The best thing you can do is to go away and try to live a normal life.' As far as he was concerned, this was positive advice, but the result was that I felt I shouldn't make any allowances for the illness. It would have been better if he'd said, 'Go away and adapt your life, get together as much support as you need in order to live the kind of life you want.' If I had been told this and been able to take it on board, I think I would have been in a better position when I embarked on motherhood four years later."

🖋 *"If I'd known more, I would have dealt with it better."*

🖋 *"Rather than just saying, 'We'll have a baby,' we decided to find out as much as possible."*

When you've been diagnosed with MS, deciding to have a baby needs careful planning. More than anything, it means being realistic about the future and the possibility that you could get worse. You have to consider whether you will be able to look after the baby yourself or whether you will need help. Plan for the worst and hope for the best.

It might be difficult to think that way when you may be only mildly affected, but if you do suffer from fatigue or walking problems later on, you'll be glad you organized the practical details in advance. It is sensible to make adjustments to the way you live. For example, if you are planning to move into a new house or apartment before the baby is born, it's wiser to choose one without too many steps and, ideally, with a toilet on the ground floor.

"Now I Curse All Those Stairs" ✿ Naomi's Story

"Thinking I would stay the same, we bought a three-story house. Now I curse all those stairs. The baby's room is at the top and the kitchen is at the bottom. Not a day goes by that I don't have to drag myself up and down the stairs to get something from the kitchen the baby needs. How I wish we'd bought an apartment instead."

Going against Other People's Attitudes

If you decide to go ahead and have a child, you may come up against negative attitudes from other people that women with a disability should not have children at all. Images still portray disabled people as victims—vulnerable, needy, and dependent—rather than as independent, powerful beings, capable of protecting and caring for other people. You may have parents, or members of your wider family, who grew up thinking that women with MS should not have children, equating disability with tragedy, shame, and even stigma for the whole family. You have to convince them that someone with MS has the same hopes and dreams as anyone else, and the same needs to have a child. You can try to win them over by telling them that new medical research, done in the 1980s and 1990s, paints a far brighter picture for mothers with MS. In the end, it's your life, and you must do what you want, despite possible opposition.

"My Mother Said, 'Just Get a Dog'" ☀ Rachel's Story

"My family was against me having a baby. They thought I would get worse. My mother said, 'Just get a dog; don't bother with a baby.' My aunt, who's a nurse, said she knew lots of patients with MS who'd gotten worse after having babies. My grandma said, 'It's not worth risking your health for a baby.' And my doctor, who knew nothing about it anyway, said, 'You don't want to change your lifestyle in case you get worse.' But we were desperate to have a child. My mother constantly brings up 'the worst case scenario' of being unable to move, in a wheelchair, and having to give my children up because I cannot care for them."

Doctors can also be insensitive to women with MS who want to have a baby, still giving out messages of doubt and anxiety about their ability to cope as mothers. Even though health professionals are far more enlightened these days than they used to be on matters of disability, it still happens that doctors make remarks such as: "I don't know whether we can allow you to have this child."[3]

The Decision Not to Have a Baby

When you have weighed all the factors you may decide against having a baby. Some women with MS—perhaps particularly those with rewarding careers—are firm in their decision not to have a child. Sometimes when a woman loves her work her whole identity is bound up with it. She earns her own money, and she may fear that having a child could jeopardize her career if her MS got worse as a result of childbearing. For some money is an important factor too. You may realistically feel you cannot afford to have a child, and that you don't have the social support you need. Others simply fear risking their own health, regardless of concerns about work or money.

"I Don't Want Anything to Put My Health At Risk" ✿ Becky's Story

"I have a career as an attorney and love what I do. Being a mother is not as important to me as being financially independent. At one time I thought I might be pregnant, and we were both relieved when I found out that I wasn't. My husband was concerned about my health, especially after hearing my neurologist say that children were a lot of work, and warned against fatigue. Having MS required me to analyze exactly who I am and what I'm about. I truly believe that I will work as long as I want to. I know my interests and my energy limitations, and my life is just what I want. I don't want anything to put my health at risk. If I got pregnant now, I would have an abortion."

"I Was Advised against Ever Getting Pregnant" ✿ Marcy's Story

"When I was diagnosed nine years ago I was advised against ever getting pregnant. They said it could worsen my MS. I was thirty at the time, and that really scared me. It definitely did put me off the idea of having children. I'm afraid that I would get worse, MS-wise, and I couldn't handle that. I'm also worried about being able to take care of a baby if I were to have one. I have a hard time using my left hand, so holding, feeding, and changing a baby would be a little difficult for me.

I'm extremely sad about not having children. All my life I have wanted children."

"Sometimes I Think Just Looking after Myself Is Enough" ☼ Alex's Story

"We're still very undecided about whether to have a baby. I think, what's my prognosis? What would it be like if I got worse? Sometimes I think just looking after myself is enough. I can rest when I want to. But when you have children, you have to put them first. I would hate any child of mine to be a caregiver. I've seen TV programs where children are caregivers for a disabled parent and I don't think children should be put in that situation. One of my greatest concerns is that we don't have enough money. I'm adamant we need adequate childcare. When I look into the future, I see us with children. But in my vision I also see a nanny and lots of money. Having no money is one of the things that really holds me back. I couldn't cope with it—it really worries me."

Emotional Consequences

Some women who have put off having a child for fear their condition would worsen feel very sad that they may not become mothers.

"I Yearn to Have a Child" ☼ Maribeth's Story

"I am thirty-four and single and have always wanted children. I put off having them just waiting for the 'right time' and the 'right relationship.' I am now struggling with the possibility that I may never become a parent. Sad is not deep enough to describe how I would feel about giving up my dreams because of the fear of a stupid disease that may or *may not* get worse. In my eyes, I would be giving up the dream of a lifetime, and I do not want to let MS take my dreams away from me too.

"I yearn to have a child and show it the beautiful things in life and to see the world through his or her unjaded eyes. I know I could be a good parent. I am patient and loving and get more joy out of being around children than anything else in my life. I have so much love to give a child. I believe there is happiness and joys that are awaiting me with children. But I am single."

Abortion (also see "Abortion" in chapter 12)

An abortion does not protect you against having a relapse. On the contrary, the relapse rate after abortions is high. In a French study of forty-nine pregnancies, eleven patients had abortions mainly or only because they suffered from MS. The reasons for the abortions varied; five women were experiencing relapses; three had taken azathioprine (which is associated with a high risk of fetal abnormalities), and three were worried about their MS worsening as a result of having a baby. The relapse rate was excessively high after the abortions.[4] In a Canadian study of fifty-three women, four had abortions. One woman was unmarried, one had no support, another woman and her husband feared having a baby could make her MS worse, and the fourth was acting on the advice of a neurologist. This woman had experienced severe relapses during three previous pregnancies and had another relapse before the fourth pregnancy could be terminated.

What the Medical Literature Says about Abortion

Pregnant patients with MS should not terminate their pregnancies solely because of their MS. There is some risk of exacerbation following termination of pregnancy at any time during gestation.[5]

The risk of relapse exists after pregnancy of any duration. Abortion and miscarriage are both followed by some increase in the risk for relapse. However the exact relapse rate has not been determined.[6]

4 ☀ Can You Stop Yourself from Getting Worse?

The decision whether to have a baby is greatly affected by the fear that MS will worsen, but this does not take into account the fact that it seems possible to stabilize or even improve your condition. Many people with MS achieve improvement by changing their diets and lifestyles. The new medications can also cut the rate of relapses and slow the progression of the disease.

"I Have Changed the Way I Eat and Live" ☀ Sandra's Story

"Slowly over the years I have changed the way I eat and live. I started seeing a naturopath and supplementing my new diet with vitamins, minerals, and evening primrose oil. I gave up dairy products and caffeine and only drink alcohol occasionally. Now I can still do everything. I take care of the children and do the household chores myself."

SOME RECOMMENDED DIETARY AND LIFESTYLE CHANGES

- Eat a diet low in saturated fat and high in unsaturated fat.

- Test for and treat candidiasis.

- Give up foods you are allergic to.

- Take nutritional supplements.

- Exercise.

- Take regular rests and naps.

- Reduce stress.

- Do some complementary therapies.

- Possibly take drug treatments for MS.

Low Saturated—and High Unsaturated—Fat Diet

Many people who have MS have found that they can effectively manage the severity of their symptoms by adhering to a diet that is very low in saturated fats. The low saturated fat diet is based on research carried out for more than forty years by Professor Roy Swank, a neurologist at the Swank MS Clinic in Portland, Oregon. During the 1940s Professor Swank looked at the distribution of MS around the world. He observed that MS is more common in countries where people eat a lot of dairy products and less common where they do not. Based on this circumstantial evidence, Swank came up with a hypothesis:

> The three-fold increase in fat intake in the past 200 years in the western world has caused a breakdown in the ability of the blood to maintain the fat and other matter in an emulsified state. The emulsion breaks down; the formed elements in the blood aggregate; and micro-embolism of the micro-circulation with consequent breakdown of the blood-brain barrier follow.[1]

Since 1951 Professor Swank has been following the cases of 150 patients with MS. He has looked at the relationship of their fat intake to their progress of disability and to the number of deaths. What he found was very clear-cut: Patients who stuck faithfully to the low-fat diet were still walking and working decades later. Those who did not stick to the diet had gotten worse, or died.[2] Professor Swank says that a low fat diet decreases the rate of exacerbation by 37 percent during the first year and halts the progression in early cases by three years. It also has no side effects.[3]

The Swank Low-Fat Diet

Although this has become known as the "low-fat diet," it really means a diet low in saturated fat but high in healthy unsaturated fat.

- Fat in meat, poultry, liver, and eggs must be kept to a minimum. Oils containing essential fatty acids (see table "Sources of Essential Fatty Acids") must be included in the quantity of at least 20 grams (four teaspoons) a day. Working, walking people could increase this to eight teaspoons, and very active people to ten teaspoons.

SOURCES OF ESSENTIAL FATTY ACIDS

Sunflower seed oil, safflower seed oil, soybean oil, corn oil, flax seed oil (linseed oil), cod liver oil, oil of evening primrose

Sunflower seeds, sesame seeds, peanuts (and peanut butter as long as it is not hydrogenated), almonds, cashew nuts

Polyunsaturated margarines

Tuna fish, salmon, sardines, herring, mackerel (see caution about canned oily fish on page 47)

Dark green leafy vegetables, such as spinach and kale

- In Dr. Swank's diet forbidden foods include:

  full-cream milk
  cream and sour cream
  butter
  ice cream
  cheese
  imitation dairy products made with palm oil (a satu-
    rated fat)
  hard margarines
  shortening
  lard
  chocolate
  cocoa butter
  coconut
  coconut and palm oils
  packaged commercial cake and cookie mixes
  potato chips
  party-type snacks
  all commercially prepared pies, cakes, pastries, dough-
    nuts and cookies
  all processed meat and poultry, luncheon meat, salami,
    frankfurters, canned meat products

- Foods that can be eaten in any quantity include:

  fish
  shellfish
  whole grain cereals and bread
  rice
  breast of poultry with the skin removed
  skimmed milk
  low-fat cottage cheese and yogurt
  clear soups
  pasta
  cornmeal
  all fresh fruits
  all fresh vegetables
  frozen or canned vegetables without butter
  jam, marmalade
  honey, sugar, molasses, corn syrup, maple syrup
  jelly
  tea, coffee
  carbonated drinks
  alcoholic drinks in moderation

How Much Fat Is "Low Fat"? Professor Swank is very strict on how much saturated fat someone with MS can safely eat. He allows only 15 grams a day—about three teaspoons. He says that if MS patients exceed this allowance even by a small amount of fat, they slowly get worse. This can happen all too easily to patients who have been stable on the low-fat diet. Once they do slip from the diet, they are unlikely to return to a stable condition. Dr. Swank warns against buying things off the supermarket shelves that give the impression of being "low in fat," but in fact are not. His regular *Swank Newsletter* gives detailed information on which American foodstuffs are allowed and which are forbidden. The newsletter is also excellent for general advice on lifestyle.

This diet is designed specifically for people who have multiple sclerosis. Even though many Americans eat too much saturated fat, it is not intended for other people.

But Is It Science? Professor Swank's research has been published in such prestigious international medical journals as *The New England Journal of Medicine,* the *American Journal of Clinical Nutrition,* and *The Lancet.* By virtue of this it has some scientific pedigree, even if some neurologists take issue with how scientific his methods are.

There are other doctors who agree that a diet low in saturated fat should be followed by people with MS. In his major reference work, *Nutritional Influences on Illness,* Melvyn R. Werbach, M.D., Assistant Clinical Professor at the UCLA School of Medicine, cites low-fat diet as the primary recommendation for MS patients.[4]

Recently, Professor Swank's hypothesis about fat and multiple sclerosis has been supported by other research. One study looked at the relationships between the mortality rates for multiple sclerosis in thirty-six countries for the period 1983–1989.[5] They examined the intake of saturated fat and the ratio of unsaturated fatty acids to saturated fat. They found a definite link between MS and high intake/high ratio of saturated fats to unsaturated fats.

The Link between Fats and MS There is clear evidence that people who have MS are low in certain essential fatty acids, especially linoleic acid. Taking more linoleic acid can make a difference to the relapse rate. This has been known since the early 1970s. Researchers of MS dietary therapy published these results in 1989.

> Analysis of blood, blood cells and cerebro-spinal fluid shows that levels of linoleic acid (LA) are lower in patients with multiple sclerosis than in healthy controls. Studies employing dietary supplementation with LA indicate a reduction in severity and length of relapses.[6]

And a 1991 article on blood analysis of MS patients stated, "Studies of membrane lipid content show that in patients with confirmed MS, cell membrane fatty acid content is abnormal."[7]

Eat a Diet High in Unsaturated Fat

Because there is such a strong link between unsaturated fat deficiency and MS, the second essential recommendation in the list of dietary and lifestyle changes is to increase the amount of unsaturated fat you eat. Generally speaking, unsaturated fats are liquid or soft at room temperature. Saturated fats are often—but not always—hard. Unsaturated fat can either be monounsaturated, as in olive oil, or polyunsaturated, as in sunflower seed oil, safflower seed oil, soya, and corn oil. Both are healthy types of fat.

Vegetable and seed oils contain something important called linoleic acid. Fish oils and certain vegetables contain alpha-linolenic acid. Both these are known as *essential fatty acids*.

They are vital to health because they convert in the body to important molecules needed for the immune system to work properly. Even if you include plenty of foods rich in essential fatty acids in your diet (see table on page 40), it is also wise to take supplements.

SUPPLEMENTS CONTAINING ESSENTIAL FATTY ACIDS

Evening primrose oil

Borage oil (also known as starflower oil)

Blackcurrant oil

Fish oils (also known as marine oils)

Eat plenty of the healthy fats and cut down—or eliminate completely—the bad fats, which have no health value, and which could do you harm.

Hydrogenated Fats Many foods are made with fats that have been heated using a process called hydrogenation. Look for "hydrogenated fat" on labels. Take peanut butter, for example. In its natural, unadulterated state, peanuts contain the healthy linoleic acid. But many brands of peanut butter are made with hydrogenated fats. Once linoleic acid is hydrogenated, it turns into a biologically different form of fat that behaves like saturated fat. What were originally biologically active essential fatty acids are turned into biologically inactive *trans fatty acids*.

Trans Fatty Acids These are fatty acids that have been stripped of their immune system enhancing properties due to food processing techniques. Far from being healthy fats, trans fatty acids compete with genuine essential fatty acids for your body's time and attention. They elbow the really good fats out of the action. The trans fatty acids that you eat make their way into tissues like the brain, heart, and lungs and may do harm. They are most commonly found in the kind of foods Americans love most—things like cookies, pastries, chips, fries, candy, and spreads.

PERCENTAGE OF TRANS FATTY ACIDS IN COMMON FOODSTUFFS[8]

Bakery products—up to 38.5 percent

Candy—up to 38.6 percent

French fries—up to 37.4 percent

Hard margarines—up to 36 percent

Soft margarines—up to 21.3 percent

Diet margarines—up to 17.9 percent

Vegetable oils—up to 13.7 percent

Cook Your Own Food Convenience foods are likely to contain trans fatty acids. The way to avoid eating fat that has lost its healthy properties is to cook your own food at home. It is more labor-intensive, but you reap the reward in health benefits (and there are cost savings as well). There are many excellent books and newsletters with healthy recipes especially for people with MS (see appendix B).

Testing and Treating for Candidiasis

Candidiasis is a yeastlike infection that interferes with normal digestion in the gut. It is caused by an abnormal bloom of the parasitic fungus *Candida albicans,* which normally resides in the mouth, vagina, and intestinal tract in much smaller and totally benign numbers. Candidiasis is common in conjunction with MS. Symptoms include chronic digestive problems such as heartburn, painful intestinal gas, bloating, diarrhea, and constipation; extreme fatigue; widespread muscular pain; and varying degrees of irritability, anxiety, or even depression. Sometimes a candida infection affects the mouth or the vagina as well, resulting in thrush or vaginitis.[9]

If you have a candida imbalance, you are likely to crave high carbohydrate, sweet foods such as cakes, cookies, candy, and pastries. Eating these only makes the problem worse. To treat candidiasis, you have to give up all sugar and sweets. Some people also find that they are sensitive to yeasted bakery products, fermented things like wine and vinegar, and mushrooms and other fungi. If you suspect candida imbalance might be a problem for you by all means have your doctor test for it. People often find that they only have to adhere to the most restrictive diet for a limited time in order to restore balance. Then they are able to reintroduce some of the offending foods in moderation.

Leaky Gut

It is common for people with MS to have leaky gut syndrome. This is a condition where incompletely digested food particles leak through permeable gut walls, causing food allergies, joint problems, and other symptoms. It can be cured through better nutrition.

Give Up Foods You Are Allergic To

The most common food allergens with MS are wheat, milk and dairy products, yeast, sugar, tea and coffee, chocolate, beef, and alcohol. You can be allergic to any food, no matter how seemingly "healthy," for example bananas, tomatoes, potatoes, citrus fruits, or apples. Fatigue is one of the most common symptoms associated with food allergies. Many people have found that when they give up the offending foods, fatigue and other MS symptoms lessen.

Take Nutritional Supplements

You may have been told that you will get all the nutrients you need from eating a healthy, balanced diet, but this may not be the case when you have MS. People with MS can have lower than normal levels of essential fatty acids. This shortfall can be made up by taking supplements of certain oils, especially evening primrose oil (or borage oil, also known as starflower oil), and either fish oils or flax seed oil (linseed oil). These oils need to be taken in conjunction with certain vitamins and minerals to be used effectively by the body, particularly vitamin C, Vitamin B_6, zinc, and magnesium. To get the right balance of oils, you need to take both gamma-linolenic acid (found in evening primrose oil and borage oil) and alpha-linolenic acid (found in either fish oils or flax seed oil). *Caution*: Recent studies have found unacceptable levels of mercury in some types of canned fish, such as tuna. Since mercury is stored in fat and is a serious teratogen, mercury levels in fish oil could be a source of concern for pregnant women. Flax seed oil imparts the same benefits as fish oil.

In addition, it is sensible to take a broad spectrum multivitamin, mineral, and trace element tablet that contains a good balance of everything, including selenium. Ideally you should have B_{12} injections as B_{12} is not absorbed well via the gut. Also add pycnogenol and grape seed extract, which are high in antioxidants, *Ginkgo biloba* and phosphatidylserine, which are good for brainpower and memory, and coenzyme Q10 and ginseng, both good for energy.*

NUTRITIONAL SUPPLEMENTS

Evening primrose oil or starflower oil (borage)
Flax seed oil (linseed oil) or fish oils
Vitamin C
Vitamin B_6
Zinc
Magnesium
Multivitamin and mineral and trace element capsule
B_{12} injections
Antioxidants (pycnogenol, grape seed extract)
Ginkgo biloba
Phosphatidylserine
Coenzyme Q10
Ginseng

Exercise

Regular exercise is an important component of a healthy lifestyle. Exercise is important because it keeps the muscles in tone, improves circulation, gives you stamina and endurance, increases flexibility, increases overall well-being, and curbs depression. It doesn't matter what kind of exercise you do, just do it frequently and consistently and get in to some kind of regular routine. If you are young and your symptoms are

---

*For fuller details, read *Multiple Sclerosis: A Self-Help Guide to Its Management* by Judy Graham (Rochester, Vt.: Healing Arts Press, 1989).

mild, you may be able to play sports, do aerobics, run, walk, ski, or swim. If your leg power is affected, you can still work out gently in a gym or on an exercise bike. If you have little strength, there are many passive exercise machines on the market designed especially for disabled people.

You may have gotten the idea that you shouldn't exercise for fear that it will wear you out. In fact, regular exercise—done properly—gives you energy. But don't overdo it. You should never exercise to the point of exhaustion. Rest when you need to, stop before you get overheated, and use a fan or air conditioning to keep cool if you are exercising indoors.

Take Regular Rests and Naps

Although exercise is important, so is rest. If you feel tired, take a rest. Don't soldier on valiantly until you are too fatigued to take another step. Rest means relaxing totally, ideally lying flat on a bed or settee, with your eyes closed, doing absolutely nothing. This helps recharge your batteries. Taking a nap is even better. Many people who take a nap in the afternoon find they wake up with enough energy to be able to do things in the evening. If you don't take a nap, you can be drained by the evening.

Reduce Stress

People with MS can be very sensitive to stress. The slightest thing can trigger tension, anxiety, worry, fear, or panic. What causes stress to one person may not to another, so you have to analyze what things cause stress in your life. Typical stressful situations include having too much to do with too little time to do it; being with people you don't like; being in situations where you feel you might be out of your depth.

One way to reduce stress is to avoid such situations, or rearrange your life to cope with them better. Say *no* more often; refuse to take on work or chores that make you feel pressured; finish one task before you start another; allow plenty of time to get places and do things; don't see people you don't like; plan things carefully. You might also like to use a relaxation technique or therapy that appeals to you, like massage, meditation, biofeedback, t'ai chi, or yoga (see "Complementary Therapies" below). Do things you enjoy, whether it's listening to music, being outside in beautiful scenery, making love, or watching your favorite programs on TV. It's easier to be relaxed if you have fun, laughter, and pleasure in your life.

Try Complementary Therapies

Thousands of people with MS turn to complementary therapies for relief of symptoms and to increase general well-being. Proponents and practitioners of complementary therapies tend to look at a person as a whole, rather than as a representative of a disease category. They also treat each person as an individual, and put the person in charge of his or her own health.

A national survey reported in the *Journal of the American Medical Association* found that use of alternative therapies increased from 33.8 percent in 1990 to 42.1 percent in 1997.[10] The therapies experiencing the greatest increases in use are herbal medicine, massage, megavitamins, self-help groups, folk remedies, energy healing, and homeopathy.

The complementary therapies most commonly practiced in the United States by people with MS are:

acupuncture and acupressure
aromatherapy
autogenic training
ayurveda
bee venom therapy
biofeedback
cannabis
chiropractic
diet and supplements
enzyme therapy
exercise
Feldenkrais
herbal medicine
homeopathy
hydrotherapy
hyperbaric oxygen
hypnotherapy
magnet therapy
massage
meditation
megavitamins
music therapy
osteopathy
polarity therapy
psychotherapy and counseling
reflexology
reiki
relaxation and guided imagery
shiatsu
t'ai chi and qigong
transcutaneous electrical nerve stimulation
traditional chinese medicine
yoga

There have been few trials on complementary therapies, so there is not much scientific data to back them up. Many people are happy to accept "anecdotal" evidence. They think: If it works for other people, maybe it will work for me too. Others want scientific evidence that a therapy works, and solid proof that it does not cause harm. There is an increasing demand for "evidence-based medicine" and trials of alternative therapies are being undertaken in university and hospital settings, using orthodox methods. Those complementary therapies for MS that have undergone some scientific testing are described below.

Acupuncture

Acupuncture helps balance the body. In the terms of traditional Chinese medicine, it balances the yin and yang. For MS, acupuncture is used to relieve pain and improve movement and sensation. Fine needles are placed at various acupuncture points along energy channels called meridians to stimulate "chi," or energy. By stimulating these points, blockages in energy flow are released. Heat or electrical stimulation can sometimes be applied at acupuncture points. One study that looked at acupuncture as a treatment for spasticity in MS found the results "encouraging enough to invite further investigation."[11]

Bee Venom Therapy

Thousands of Americans with MS have tried bee venom therapy (BVT). Based on the widely-publicized successes of individuals like "Bee Lady" Pat Wagner of Maryland and Donna Domby of Michigan, people have flown to these women's homes to be stung by bees. On average, they get twenty-five to thirty honeybee stings per session and average more than three thousand stings per year. Supporters claim the bee venom therapy helps with walking, numbness, fatigue, and other MS symptoms.

Honeybee venom contains a mixture of toxins and biologically active compounds that may be anti-inflammatory. As there may be a potential benefit for MS, studies are in progress. A preliminary trial at Allegheny University of the

Health Sciences in Philadelphia on mice with the MS-like disease EAE found that honeybee venom had no beneficial effect against the disease, and some of the mice treated with bee venom got worse.[12] But they felt more research was needed. Now BVT is undergoing scientific tests at Georgetown University Medical Center in Washington, DC, thanks to a grant from the Multiple Sclerosis Society of America. The phase 1 study is examining the safety and tolerance of honeybee venom extracts as a possible therapy for MS. It will aim to provide a scientific basis for dosage, and discover potential side effects. If successful, a full-scale trial will follow.

Important Caution: Bee stings can cause life-threatening allergic reactions. The National Multiple Sclerosis Society recommends waiting until further tests are done to see if it is safe, and if it works.

Biofeedback

Biofeedback is a well-established method of dealing with stress, but it can also be used to improve ataxia (unsteady gait and staggering walk) in MS. Patients use a monitoring machine to help them control physiological processes like blood pressure. A German study found a significant improvement in ataxia using biofeedback techniques.[13]

Cannabis

Many people with MS who use cannabis claim that it helps treat spasticity, muscle spasm, pain, tremor, staggering walk, and poor balance. Anecdotal reports have inspired several small trials, and more are in the pipeline both in the United States and in Europe. One study on the active ingredient of cannabis, delta-9-THC (tetrahydrocannabinol), found a significant improvement in MS patient ratings of spasticity compared to placebo.[14] The patients also felt "high." Another trial found that cannabis reduced spasticity, rigidity, and pain, resulting in improved mobility.[15] So far, the trials on cannabis have not been rigorous enough to satisfy medical scientists as to its effectiveness and long-term safety. Marijuana still remains a controlled agent under current policies of the U.S. Drug Enforcement Agency. *Caution:* Cannabis should not be taken by pregnant women or nursing mothers.

Diet

Many people with MS have changed their diet so that they eat more unsaturated fat and less saturated fat. The effectiveness of this dietary change is backed up by several scientific studies. The general conclusion is that exacerbations are shorter and less severe in patients eating a high amount of unsaturated fats and a small amount of saturated fat.[16, 17] One researcher, Dr. Robert Dworkin, found that "[dietary] treatment reduced the severity and duration of relapses at all levels of disability and duration of illness at entry to the trials."[18]

Evening Primrose Oil

The supplement most frequently used by people with MS is evening primrose oil. This oil is high in linoleic acid and GLA (gamma-linolenic acid), which converts into prostaglandin E_1, a molecule that is anti-inflammatory and helps regulate the immune system. The dose needs to be high enough to have any effect.[19] An effective dose would be twelve 500 mg capsules per day, divided up so that you take four with each meal. Evening primrose oil should be taken with vitamin E. Flax seed oil (or fish oils) should also be taken to give a balance of essential fatty acids. Many other supplements are used by people with MS, but these have not undergone clinical trials specifically for MS.

Exercise

The benefits of exercise for MS patients have been tested at the University of Washington. A study carried out by exercise scientists Alan Alquist and George H. Kraft[20] treated eight cases of MS using progressive resistance exercise (PRE). Eight women with MS who took part in the study exercised three times a week under careful supervision. Each session consisted of stretching and performing three sets of exercise repetitions for each muscle group. The results were positive. Gains in peak strength were observed in all muscle groups, although the gains in strength were greater for those with mild MS. The patients could also walk faster, climb steps more easily, and perform strength tests better after doing PRE. The researchers concluded that PRE training for people with MS improves the ability to perform common daily activities, has a positive psychosocial effect, strengthens muscles, and improves overall well-being.

Homeopathy

Homeopathy is based on the principle that "like cures like." It uses highly dilute remedies. A homeopath looks at the whole person, including personality and lifestyle, before choosing remedies tailor-made to the individual. One author lists fifty-six homeopathic remedies that could be used in the treatment of MS.[21] There are case reports of improvements in MS symptoms in people who were given homeopathic treatment.[22] But this does not amount to hard scientific evidence and there are only cautiously positive conclusions for homeopathy in the treatment of MS.[23]

Magnet Therapy

Magnet therapy can help improve many MS symptoms: bladder control, cognitive function, fatigue, mobility, spasticity, and vision. In a double-blind study, thirty MS patients were exposed to a magnetic pulsing device (Enermed). They wore the device on preselected sites between ten and twenty-four hours a day for two months. The magnetic device demonstrated a statistically significant effect.[24]

Massage and Aromatherapy

Massage, in all its various forms, is a very popular therapy for MS. It is relaxing, relieves stress and tension, and is pleasurable. Research has also found that it lowers anxiety and depression, raises self-esteem, and gives people a general sense of well-being.[25] There are anecdotal reports of improvements in self-image of individuals with MS who have had massage.[26] Also, a pilot study where ten patients were stroked for three minutes at a time made them feel more relaxed.[27]

Psychotherapy and Counseling

Being told you have MS is traumatic. Psychotherapy or counseling can help you adjust to the condition, manage associated depression or anxiety, and can boost self-esteem. One study that looked at the benefits of group psychotherapy on patients with MS found it significantly reduced depression and improved emotional state.[28]

Reflexology

In reflexology certain zones of the feet are stimulated by a practitioner. These zones relate to specific organs and parts of the body. Reflexology is particularly helpful for bladder problems, but can also improve motor and sensory symptoms. In a clinical trial, seventy-one MS patients were studied. Half were given reflexology, the other half a dummy treatment. Both groups were tested for numbness, bladder problems, muscle strength, and spasticity. The results showed a significant improvement in the group given reflexology.[29]

Relaxation and Guided Imagery

Helping MS patients use guided imagery can bring about a significant reduction in anxiety and can imporve patients' perceptions of their illness. A study on thirty-three patients with MS in a Pennsylvania hospital found that patients given daily relaxation and guided imagery felt far less anxious than they had prior to the study.[30]

Transcutaneous Electrical Nerve Stimulation (TENS)

Lower-limb muscle-tone problems are common in patients with MS, due to increase or decrease in tone, or intermittent spasm. Thirteen percent of people with MS have painful muscle spasm that disturbs sleep.[31] This type of MS pain can be treated by placing a TENS machine on the affected area. TENS produces a significant improvement in symptoms both by reducing pain and frequency of spasm as well as by reducing sleep disturbance. Improvement in symptoms is seen in 75 percent of patients.[32] The TENS machine should be used over the affected muscle groups for a minimum of eight hours a day for at least two weeks. TENS has the advantages of being relatively cheap, easy to use, and without the side effects of medication.

"By Living Strangely in the Eyes of Others . . . I Keep Going" ✺ John Pageler's Story

"I'm sure a strict low-fat diet, the right kind of supplements, the right type of exercise, and the correct mental attitude would keep many more MS patients walking and working. Now, with the help of my exercise program, magnet therapy, and massage, I'm able to walk short distances and mow the lawn. I could have been 100 percent disabled by now. But instead I live a productive life, play tennis, run my own business, and travel the world.

"I'm looking for a better quality of life! By living strangely in the eyes of others—that is, eating weird, exercising daily, keeping a positive mental attitude—I keep going with good energy and cognitive ability. Sure I have problems that come and go, but I'm sure the reason they come and go, instead of putting me down, is my willingness to do what needs to be done to control my MS."

Drug Treatments for MS: Betaseron, Avonex, and Copaxone

🖝 *"I started on Betaseron, which I took for two years, and then have been on Avonex ever since. I have not had a major exacerbation since 1993."*

🖝 *"Since I was put on Betaseron, I haven't had an attack. I still have leg weakness, and my bladder never went back to normal, but I have learned to live with that."*

"The MS has stopped dead in its tracks. Avonex hasn't cured me, but I haven't gotten any worse."

These new drugs reduce the frequency of relapses. Avonex can also slow down the progression of the disease. Some people with MS do very well on them, experiencing markedly fewer attacks. Others find the side effects unpleasant enough that they decide to stop taking drugs. The most common side effects are flulike symptoms and inflammation at the site of injection. These tend to lessen over time, so it is probably worth giving these drugs a fair trial before giving up. Your doctor will be able to prescribe the appropriate dose for you.

As these drugs are quite new, they have not been tested on MS people over a prolonged length of time, so no one knows the long-term side effects. (See chapter 7 for more information about drug treatments.)

5 ✸ Relationships, Sexuality, and Fertility

If you are disabled with MS, it can make forming relationships much harder. You may feel self-conscious about the way you look, and going out to meet people can be problematic. But there are many people who are not put off by disability, and there are plenty of other disabled people longing to meet someone. Forming a close relationship fulfills a basic human need. As with all other aspects of life, MS should not prevent you from doing this. You may need help from a therapist in changing your inner feelings and low self-esteem.

🖋 *"I do think MS is part of why I am not married. It's hard to meet people and date when you walk with a walker, live with your parents, and have no way to meet people. I would like to think that if it were not for MS, I would be married with children."*

MS—A Severe Test of a Relationship

Having MS can be a severe test of a relationship. Many men and women relate that their relationships fell apart when they told a partner they had MS. It can be a painful experience. Once this has happened, the person with MS can feel grateful to anyone who shows an interest, which is no basis for a relationship. On the other hand, some partners rise to the challenge and show what terrific human beings they are. These are the ones who want to make life wonderful for the man or woman who has MS. Luckily, there are plenty of terrific human beings around.

🌿 *"When I told Steve I had MS he told me, 'Let's get married straightaway.' I knew then that he really loved me."*

🌿 *"I think I married my husband partly out of panic. A man had broken up with me just prior to me meeting my husband. The reason: my MS. Not exactly life-affirming. I felt like damaged goods. I wondered who in the world would want me?"*

🌿 *"On my third date with Rachel, she told me she had MS. My response was to go straight to the library and educate myself about the condition. I knew that I could cope."*

Keeping a Relationship Strong

Having MS can change you. It can make you less active and possibly less attractive. It can take deep commitment and love to sustain a relationship when one partner is physically deteriorating. Hold on to your self-esteem—you are still you. Keep the communication open and loving. If it gets to be a bumpy ride, both of you may need counseling or therapy.

🌿 *"Elena is not the woman I married. When I met her, she was vivacious, energetic, independent, fun, and full of laughter. Now she is dependent on me for everything, lethargic, and a misery."*

Sexuality and MS

MS does not lessen the need for loving, sexual relationships, but it can alter the sexual response in both men and women.

Sexual Problems in Women

There is little research on sexual problems in women with MS. From the little data we have, however, it seems that in at least 56 percent of cases, MS can bring on sexual difficulties. Even so, many women with MS can find pleasure once they are engaged in sexual intercourse, and—with an open attitude—there are several ways to overcome problems. Common problems are lower libido, difficulty with arousal, decreased sensation in the genital and other regions, more difficulty in reaching orgasm or loss of orgasm, fatigue that interferes with sex, and problems with vaginal lubrication. Women with bladder problems can fear wetting the bed during sex or are embarrassed by wearing a catheter. For women with spastic movements, getting into different positions can also be a problem.

Some of these problems are caused by damage in the spinal cord, but they can be complicated by psychological causes. Women may feel less attractive and less sexy because of MS, especially if they use disability aids like walkers or wheelchairs. MS symptoms may also make them feel less vivacious. This change in self-image can make them depressed, and they can suffer loss of self-esteem. Such feelings can inhibit sexual desire and increase feelings of anxiety and vulnerability. Depression can also lower libido.

Solutions to Sexual Problems in Women

With a loving partner, open and honest communication, real intimacy, and the kind of attitude that says, do whatever works, many problems can be overcome. Here are a few solutions.

- Lubricants like KY Jelly can help with decreased vaginal lubrication.

- Vibrators can give more intense stimulation to bring a woman to orgasm.

- Viagra increases blood flow to the genital area and makes orgasm easier. It was designed for men, but it works on women too.

- If fatigue is an issue, set aside a time for sex when you are least tired. Sex does not have to be vigorous to be satisfying.

- If particular positions are difficult, experiment with others.

- Depression can be treated with herbal remedies such as St. John's wort.

- Spasticity can be treated with medication.

- Bladder and bowel dysfunction can be treated with medication. If incontinence is a problem, cut down on drinks before intercourse. Empty the bowel and bladder before intercourse. If a catheter has to be worn, it can be taped out of the way.

- Create a romantic setting for lovemaking, using sensual music, lighting, and so forth.

• Devote time to nurturing your relationship. It is essential to maintain intimacy.

Sexual Problems in Men

MS can make fatherhood difficult to achieve because any disturbance in erection can make intercourse and ejaculation impossible; for women, sex is still possible despite loss of feeling. It has been estimated that up to 91 percent of men with MS suffer from erection dysfunction at some time in the course of the disease, although emotional factors are thought to play a part. About 25 percent of men with MS do become impotent, but this symptom, like others, can remit. Sexual symptoms in men can range from minor difficulties in gaining and maintaining an erection to disturbances of sensation and ejaculation to total failure to achieve an erection. Ejaculation may be affected because it is controlled by the bundle of nerves in the lower spinal cord. Men who have difficulty getting or maintaining an erect penis may be less likely to ejaculate. Like women, men with MS can also suffer from diminished sensation and libido, bladder and bowel problems, and feelings of loss of masculinity and self-esteem. These problems can be treated similarly to how they are handled for women.

Ways to Treat Impotence

Viagra The newest impotence therapy is the drug Viagra, which is being tested specifically for MS at the time of this writing. It is known to be effective in about 70 percent of cases of erectile dysfunction in men with such conditions as spinal cord injury and diabetes. There is no reason why Viagra should not work just as well in MS. One Viagra tablet should be taken an hour or so before lovemaking. It works by targeting a specific enzyme produced in the penis during sexual stimulation. This has the effect of relaxing erectile muscle and boosting the blood supply to the penis. As it fills with blood, the penis becomes erect, and the effect lasts as long as sexual stimulation continues. Side effects can include headaches, facial flushing, indigestion, and a stuffy nose. There have also been some reports of Viagra causing heart problems in patients with preexisting heart conditions.

Injecting Medications A medication is injected into the base of the penis, which gives it an erection. The injection is done with a very fine needle or with an "auto-injector," which works with a simple push-button mechanism. It is not as painful as it sounds. Prostaglandin E_1 (alprostadil, also known as Prostin VR) is the drug most commonly used in MS. This substance is a vasodilator and smooth-muscle relaxant, similar to the natural substance released by the smooth-muscle cells in the penis when a man is sexually excited. Relaxation of smooth muscle in the penis prevents blood from leaving the penis once it enters, allowing for erection to occur. Other injection-type drugs are papaverine and phentolamine (Regitine). Phentolamine is sometimes used in combination with prostaglandin E_1 and/or papaverine to heighten their effectiveness.

Urethral Suppositories In the United States, prostaglandin E_1 is also available via urethral suppository, which can be used instead of penile injections. A small plastic applicator inserts the drug into the urethra. The drug is absorbed into penile tissues and stimulates an erection. Slight discomfort, prolonged erections (priapism), and scarring at the site of injection can sometimes result with these injections and urethral suppositories.

Vacuum Erection Devices (VEDs) These devices consist of vacuum tubes and constriction bands. With the VED, a plastic tube is fitted over the flaccid penis, and a hand pump or suction tube is operated to create a vacuum. The vacuum draws blood into the erectile tissues and produces an erection. Once engorgement of the penis takes place, a latex band is slipped from the cylinder onto the base of the penis. This band maintains engorgement of the penis by restricting venous return of blood to the body, thus allowing for sexual activity. This method has several disadvantages. The use of the band must be limited to thirty minutes to avoid complications, quite good hand sensation and dexterity are needed to put it on and take it off, and bruising and nipping of the skin are common. Despite these caveats, patient and partner satisfaction with this method is high.

Penile Prosthesis A penile prosthesis is a surgically implanted mechanical device that is designed to give a man with erectile dysfunction the option of having an erection. There are two types: semirigid and inflatable. With the semirigid type, a flexible rod is implanted by a urological surgeon in each of the erection chambers of the penis. Being flexible, these rods can be bent upward when an erection is desired and downward at other times. Once the rods are inserted, the penis remains somewhat enlarged with a permanent semierection.

With the inflatable type, a fluid is pumped from a reservoir into balloons inserted in the penis, resulting in an erection. The reservoir is surgically implanted behind the abdominal wall, and the pump is implanted in the man's scrotum. Complications can sometimes arise. This surgery is generally used only when more noninvasive methods have been tried unsuccessfully.

"It's a Bit of a Delicate Procedure" ☀ John's Story

"I was impotent for two years. I just couldn't get an erection. Then I found a specialist who gave me a drug that you inject into your penis. It is a bit of a delicate procedure, but you get the hang of it. You have to be careful not to inject too much, or you're left with an erection for hours and you have to go to the hospital for an antidote. When my wife got pregnant, I did wonder at first whether it was mine. I thought she might have found an outlet for her sexual needs elsewhere. But now I'm sure the baby is mine."

Is Fertility Affected by MS?

🖋 *"It took fourteen months to get pregnant. We decided we'd just let nature take its course. We weren't exactly going hammer and tong, but when I still wasn't pregnant after thirteen months I did start to worry about my fertility. And then I got pregnant. We were so happy."*

🖋 *"God knows how I got pregnant! I was using contraceptives, was seeing my partner only once every three weeks, and was thirty-seven years old. My son must have had a very strong will to be born!"*

The fact that fewer women with MS have babies than the rest of the female population does not mean that they are less fertile, and there is nothing to show that MS affects fertility as such. In general, the number of pregnancies among women with MS is not different from the rate in control groups. One research study did show an apparent reduction in fertility of

13 percent. There may be several reasons for this statistic. Some women with MS, particularly if it is severe, deliberately decide not to have a baby because of fears that their condition will worsen. Some are advised by their doctors against getting pregnant.

Indeed, some women with MS may decide not to get married or do not have the same chances of marriage, and these women are unlikely to have children. Divorce rates are higher among patients who are more severely disabled. Women with MS also tend to have fewer children. Women whose symptoms worsened after having one child may be unlikely to have another child. In addition, women with MS have more elective abortions, and more of them undergo sterilization.

Miscarriage

The rate of spontaneous abortions, congenital malformations, or stillbirths among women with MS is not higher than the rate for the general population.

6 ✸ Pregnancy and Prenatal Care

In the six months before conception, you—and your partner —should aim to stay as healthy as possible. Good preconceptual care can make a big difference not only to your own wellbeing during pregnancy, but also to the normal development of your baby. It optimizes the health of sperm, ova, and uterus. Such conditions as subfertility, miscarriage, low birth weight, premature birth, hyperactivity, learning problems, asthma, and eczema are to a great extent preventable by good nutrition and treating allergies, candidiasis, malabsorption, and infections before you even get pregnant. Ideally, both of you should:

- **Eat a healthy diet** (see chapter 4). You are much more likely to feel well and stay well if you stick to a healthy diet. For anyone with MS, this ideally means a diet low in animal and saturated fats, high in polyunsaturated fats, and with plenty of green leafy vegetables, fresh oily fish, liver, lean meat, poultry, legumes, and fruit. You can safely stay on this diet before getting pregnant, during pregnancy, and after the baby is born. Cut right down on junk foods and avoid additives. Buy organic when possible. Drink bottled or filtered water.

- **Give up smoking, alcohol, and drugs.** These social poisons should ideally be given up for at least four months before conception. Cigarettes, alcohol, and street drugs can have a bad effect on a fetus. They need to be cleared out of the system before getting pregnant.

- **Treat food allergies, candidiasis, and leaky gut.** (See chapter 4 for details.)

- **Use noninvasive contraception.** The contraceptive pill lowers a woman's level of zinc, manganese, vitamin A, and the B-complex vitamins. The copper IUD has effects on mineral status. A diaphragm is a noninvasive method.

- **Treat urogenital and other infections.** Both partners should be checked out for common infections such as chlamydia and herpes.

- **Get tested for unacceptable levels of heavy metals and environmental toxins.** If found, these can be removed by nutritional therapy.

In addition, the woman should:

- **Take folic acid supplements.** This is a B vitamin that helps protect against spina bifida and other neural tube defects in a baby. It should be taken both before conception and for three months into the pregnancy.

- **Engage in some gentle exercise.** Yoga and stretching exercises are particularly good during pregnancy. They increase suppleness and stretch the ligaments. You will also be fitter, more flexible, and have better muscle tone. Exercise gives you more energy. It also increases strength and endurance. All this will help during childbirth and beyond. And, if you have exercised well during pregnancy, your body will be able to "open up" more easily during childbirth.

- **Stop certain medications before getting pregnant.** (See chapter 7, "Effects of Medications for MS.")

Prenatal Care

🖝 *"During my pregnancy I wasn't treated differently from anyone else. The MS was in my notes, and they were aware of it, but that's all."*

In most cases, there is no reason why you should not be treated like any other woman in terms of prenatal care. MS does not make you a high risk patient in obstetric terms. Even so, you should certainly let the obstetric team know that you have MS and make sure that it is noted in your chart. If the doctors know you have MS and experience mobility or bladder problems, they may deal with you more delicately and sensitively.

Your Nutritional Status

Eating a healthy diet during pregnancy increases your chances of having a healthy baby. Nutrition is especially important about the time of conception and the first twelve weeks of pregnancy, because this is the time when fetal cells divide most rapidly and vital organs are developing. It is up to you to prepare the healthiest environment possible in which your unborn baby will grow. The focus on nutrition in pregnancy has tended to concentrate on protein and carbohydrates. But it is now known that the fetus, as well as a newborn baby, needs what are known as essential fatty acids.

Essential Fatty Acids Essential fatty acids are the building blocks of the brain and central nervous system. They are vital for a baby's healthy development. The placenta, through which the baby receives nutrients, also needs these fatty acids. Foods containing essential fatty acids include oily fish; green leafy vegetables; and seed oils, such as sunflower oil, safflower oil, and evening primrose oil (see tables in chapter 4 for dietary and supplemental sources of essential fatty acids). You should be very careful about the amount of foods you eat made with processed fats. Trans fatty acids, found in a wide range of manufactured foods, cross the placenta and are inhibitors of fetal growth. Scientific research into early human development has concluded that a specific profile of membrane lipids and their fatty acids is essential for normal brain integrity and functioning.[3] The same researchers note, "Essential fatty acids are important constituents of all cell membranes especially those in the brain and nervous systems."[4]

Other Nutrients Other important nutrients to include in your diet are plenty of protein and complex carbohydrates, as well as several vitamins and minerals, especially the B vitamins, magnesium, zinc, and iron. Eat lots of fresh fruits and vegetables, and take supplemental vitamins, minerals, and trace elements.

Exercise

Gentle, yoga-type exercise will help keep you supple and in good shape. Swimming is also good exercise for pregnant women.

Minor Problems during Pregnancy

You are likely to have the same minor problems during pregnancy as any other woman. None of them is usually severe enough to affect your decision to have a baby. With MS, however, particular problems can arise.

Constipation

This can be a symptom women experience as part of MS. Iron tablets taken during pregnancy can make it worse. Constipation can be treated by stool softeners, eating enough fiber, and drinking plenty of water. Prune juice is both a stool softener and an excellent source of iron.

Urinary Tract Infections

MS and pregnancy are both associated with an increase in urinary tract infections, which should be treated promptly. In some cases they can lead to pyelonephritis—a bacterial infection of the kidney that is a serious complication during pregnancy. The infection can be treated effectively with intravenous antibiotics, which do not affect the fetus.

Fatigue

Fatigue is another symptom that can be part of both MS and pregnancy. You may need to alter your lifestyle so that you can rest more.

Gait Problems

Toward the end of pregnancy, gait can worsen. With MS, poor balance and a staggering walk mean you are more likely to fall for no apparent reason, even in the safety of your own home. Make sure you always have something secure to grab on to, sturdy pieces of furniture around the home, and if necessary, a cane or a walker outside.

7 ✺ Effects of Medications for MS

As a general rule, no medications should be taken during pregnancy since they could affect the fetus. In some cases, however, doctors think it is better to take medication to treat MS, even during pregnancy. The most sensitive time for drugs to harm a fetus is in the first twelve weeks of a pregnancy. If you are taking any drugs, it is important not to get pregnant accidentally. Always discuss what medication you should take with your doctor.

Betaseron, Avonex, and Copaxone

Betaseron, Avonex, and Copaxone are the first real drug treatments targeted specifically at MS. In general, the interferon drugs, Betaseron and Avonex, decrease the relapse rate by about a third, prolong the time between relapses, and lessen their severity. Avonex also slows the progression of disability. Copaxone reduces the frequency of relapses.

Some women do well on these medications. Others stop taking them because of side effects such as flulike symptoms and inflammation at the site of injection. You may prefer to follow the holistic treatments outlined in chapter 4 as an alternative to taking these medications. Or you could combine both, as some women do successfully.

Go on the Treatment? Or Have a Baby?

With the option of taking medication that can help MS, young women are faced with a dilemma—to start the treatment first or have a baby first. Some women have a baby and then go on a medication when the baby is born. Others start on medication as soon as they can, raising the question of when they should stop if they want to have a baby. As a result, these medications are having an impact on when women with MS have a baby. They are also affecting how many children women have and whether or not they breast-feed.

Doctors advise against taking these drugs if you are trying to get pregnant. The current recommendation by the manufacturers is that one should avoid pregnancy while taking these medications. Doctors Kathy Birk and Richard Rudick concur. They say, "We would not advise any woman taking Betaseron to plan to be pregnant while taking the drug. Since exacerbation is unlikely during pregnancy, stopping Betaseron is a reasonable approach."

Fertility, Miscarriage, and Birth Defects All these drugs have been tested on animals. They had no apparent effect on fertility. When Betaseron was given to monkeys at almost three times the human dose, it did cause spontaneous abortions, suggesting a risk of birth defects. Whether a link can be made to humans is not known. There are no adequate or well-controlled studies in pregnant women.

What the Drug Companies Say about Having a Baby

Betaseron Betaseron is a registered trademark of Berlex Laboratories. *What It Is and What It Does:* Interferon beta-1b. Treatment for patients with relapsing/remitting MS who are able to walk. Reduces frequency of attacks by a third.

General Advice to Patients about Pregnancy (from Berlex Laboratories): "Betaseron should not be used during pregnancy or if you are trying to become pregnant. If you wish to become pregnant and you are using Betaseron, discuss the matter with your doctor. While using Betaseron, women of childbearing age should use birth control measures. If you do become pregnant you should discontinue treatment and contact your doctor immediately."[1]

Avonex Avonex is a registered trademark of Biogen, Inc. *What It Is and What It Does:* Interferon beta-1a. Different from Betaseron. Reduces the frequency of attacks and slows the progression of physical disability.

General Advice to Patients about Pregnancy (from Biogen, Inc.): "Avonex should not be used if you are pregnant or if you are trying to become pregnant. Women of childbearing age should use birth control during treatment with Avonex. If you want to become pregnant while being treated with Avonex, discuss the matter with your doctor. If you should become pregnant while using Avonex, stop the treatment and contact your doctor right away."[2]

Copaxone Copaxone is a registered trademark of Teva Pharmaceuticals. *What It Is and What It Does:* Copaxone (previously known as copolymer-1) is not like the interferon drugs. It is made of glatiramer acetate, a chemical that modulates the immune system. It appears to block the autoimmune attack on myelin—the fatty sheath around nerves, which is damaged in MS. It reduces the rate of relapses in patients with relapsing/remitting MS. Because Copaxone is well tolerated, it is especially suitable for patients who cannot take Betaseron or Avonex because of their side effects.

General Advice to Patients about Pregnancy (from Teva Pharmaceuticals): "Reproduction studies have been performed in rats and rabbits at doses approximately 18 to 36 times the human dose and have revealed no evidence of impaired fertility or harm to the fetus. There are, however, no adequate and well-controlled studies in pregnant women. Because animal reproduction studies are not always predictive of human response, this drug should be used during pregnancy only if clearly needed. It is important for women taking Copaxone to inform their physician if they become pregnant or plan to become pregnant. Preclinical and clinical studies show no adverse effects on reproductive ability."[3]

Other Medications

Prednisolone

This is a steroid drug that reduces inflammation during a flare-up. The chances of a bad relapse are minimized during pregnancy, and for this reason, a woman is unlikely to need steroid drugs. If your physician considers them necessary during pregnancy to stabilize severe exacerbations, they are given only in the lowest dose possible.

Steroids can pose a risk of birth defects or virilization of female fetuses if taken in the first twelve weeks of pregnancy. There is a risk of fetal adrenal suppression if corticosteroids are given at high doses late in pregnancy. In a German study,[4] three women had been treated with corticosteroids or azathioprine early in pregnancy, but none of the fetuses showed any malformations and all developed normally.

Imuran (Azathioprine) and Cyclosporine

These are immunosuppressive drugs. They should not be taken during pregnancy. Some fetal abnormalities have been reported with azathioprine taken during the first twelve weeks of pregnancy. One study on the risks of azathioprine found a high rate of fetal adverse events.[5] Four of forty-four infants had major congenital abnormalities, and 45 percent were born prematurely. In a French study,[6] three patients who had been treated with azathioprine during their pregnancies had normal babies and normal deliveries. In the same study, three other women who had been on azathioprine decided to have abortions because of their fear of birth defects. Cyclosporine may interfere with the growth of the unborn baby and also imparts a higher risk of premature birth. There is an association between the use of immunosuppressive drugs and cervical and other cancers. Any woman treated with these drugs should have regular pap tests and breast examinations.

Valium (Diazepam)

This drug is a muscle relaxant. It should be avoided during pregnancy, particularly in the first twelve weeks. It has been associated with birth defects such as cleft palate and floppy infant syndrome, and with neonatal withdrawal.

Lioresal (Baclofen) and Dantrium (Dantrolene Sodium)

These drugs treat chronic severe spasticity of voluntary muscles. Their use should be avoided during pregnancy. The manufacturer of baclofen advises that toxicity to the fetus has been noted in animal studies. Baclofen has not been shown to cause birth defects in humans. Even so, exercise caution and use this drug only if your doctor thinks it is absolutely necessary.

Oxybutynin and Propantheline

These medications are used to control bladder urgency, frequency of urination, or incontinence. Both should be discontinued before conception. They may be used only during the last six months of pregnancy if bladder problems are very exhausting for the mother.

Drugs for Epilepsy

Some people with MS also have epilepsy and need to take drugs to control it. If possible, these drugs should be stopped during pregnancy because they do raise the chance of having a malformed baby, particularly with cleft lip and palate. The risk rises to 7 percent compared with 2 percent for people not taking these drugs. Since epileptic seizures can cause damage to both the mother and baby, however, you may need to stay on a low dose in order to prevent or minimize attacks.

Vitamin, Mineral, and Other Supplements

Be particularly careful not to take too much vitamin A, since this supplement can harm the baby. Normal amounts of vitamins, minerals, trace elements, and amino acids are safe, as are evening primrose oil, fish oils (but see caution on page 47), and flax seed oil.

Hyperbaric Oxygen (HBO)

It is safer to stop sessions of HBO when you are pregnant.

Antidepressants

Medications for depression should be avoided. Manufacturers advise antidepressants should only be used if necessary. They do not cause birth defects.

St. John's Wort

Even though this is a mild herbal treatment for depression, caution is still called for. Four doctors writing in the *Journal of the American Medical Association* say: "We caution against the use of St. John's wort during pregnancy."[7]

Herbal Remedies

Herbal remedies are considered safe because they are natural. However, this may not always follow. The *Journal of the American Medical Association* says: "Clinicians should dispel the concept that if something is 'natural,' it automatically is safe. . . . Because some herbal products may cause premature uterine contractions and cross the placental barrier, use during pregnancy and by lactating women should be avoided."[8]

8 ☀ Labor and Childbirth

Women with MS can have a wide variety of birth experiences —just like anyone else. How good or bad it is usually has very little to do with MS and more to do with the physician who attends your birth, the hospital and its staff, and the way they do things there.

☛ *"The doctor was very good. He said, 'Don't worry—your body knows just what to do.'"*

☛ *"The doctor did suggest an epidural, but that was more to do with help if I got tired pushing rather than pain relief."*

☛ *"I had a suction delivery because I found it difficult to push."*

☛ *"The birth was very easy and fast—only three hours and four minutes. It was wonderful and didn't really hurt at all."*

☛ *"During the second pregnancy, I was in a wheelchair all the time. But for the labor I just got on the bed. It was very quick and all over in six hours."*

☛ *"The birth was so fast I had her in the Emergency Room. She just dropped out."*

☛ *"My first birth got a little high tech because there was fetal distress and I ended up with a monitor on the baby's head. I think the MS was immaterial."*

Labor management requires no change in routine. Analgesia where needed should be used. There is no evidence that patients with MS require or would benefit from shortening the second stage of labor. Maternal exhaustion may necessitate an instrument-assisted vaginal delivery in some cases. Cesarian section should be used only for the usual obstetric indications.[1]

Delivery is not more complicated in MS patients, and the mode of delivery is decided strictly on obstetrical criteria.[2]

🖎 *"At the end I didn't have the strength to push him out. I had a forceps delivery with an episiotomy. That was painful."*

🖎 *"My second birth was a piece of cake. I'd been doing pre-natal yoga, which was very nice and gentle. I gave birth on the bathroom floor. She was a tiny little thing. At the time, I was on a low-fat diet. The doctors said, 'You have a very small and very healthy baby.'"*

Choices in Childbirth

Even with MS, you should have the same choices about child-birth as any other woman. Today, obstetricians are more likely to take this attitude than they did even a decade ago. The muscle weakness common in MS need not affect giving birth. The birth process is all to do with hormonal balance and uterine muscles. The muscles of the uterus are smooth muscles, unlike peripheral muscles, which come under the control of the central nervous sytem. The contractions of the uterus are reflex actions. When a woman is not interfered with and not disturbed during labor, she is able to secrete the right hormones. Among them are endorphins, which give a woman a feeling of well-being and help make childbirth a joyful event.

Women with lower-limb weakness or sensory symptoms may have some difficulty pushing the baby out at the end and may need extra help. In such cases, doctors are likely to monitor the labor very carefully and use techniques to help deliver the baby safely, such as episiotomy and forceps or vacuum extraction. Another way to help delivery is to give birth in the supported squatting position, in which someone holds your shoulders, giving an upward lift. Gravity helps the baby drop down.

Should You Be Treated as a Special Case?

Try to find an obstetrician who is comfortable with MS and knows something about it. And find a neurologist who is comfortable with your being pregnant. It helps if the two of them get along and communicate. You should let your doctors know you have MS so that you can have a little extra help from hospital staff once the baby is born, if you need it. While you do not necessarily want to be thought of as different from other pregnant women, you do not want your special needs to be overlooked either.

🖎 *"My obstetrician asked me whether I wanted to be special. I said I wanted to be treated like anyone else, and that's what he did."*

🌿 "The OB/GYN never treated me differently from any other pregnant woman. I delivered a healthy seven-pound, eleven-ounce baby boy."

🌿 "Most of the medical staff I dealt with were totally uninterested about my multiple sclerosis and left me to my own devices. I was very anxious, since my body was totally numb until two weeks before the birth—so I never felt the baby kick or move. So the 'kick chart' I was given was a joke! When I was totally paralyzed for twelve hours three days after the birth, the nurses panicked, suddenly realizing that I wasn't a 'normal' mom and that I really did need help."

"The Hospital Staff Did Almost Nothing to Help Me"
✹ Rachel's Story

"My husband, Mark, had to be my nurse because the hospital staff did almost nothing to help me. He was the one who gave me a bath after the baby was born. He was the one who helped me down from the bed so I could feed the baby. The hospital bed was so high, I couldn't get down on my own. I was in tears. Mark had to do everything for me and virtually moved in to the hospital. Some days I was too weak to get out of bed and stand in the queue for breakfast. The nurses wouldn't have brought it to me. One nurse on night duty was really unpleasant. She said, 'Why are you bothering me with problems with breast-feeding?'"

Natural Childbirth

There is no reason why a woman with MS cannot have a normal vaginal delivery. Dr. Kathy Birk encourages natural childbirth for women with MS.

You need to have the freedom to find the most comfortable birthing position. It could be on all fours, kneeling, semisquatting, squatting while holding on to something or someone, standing, leaning, lunging forward, sitting, or lying down. An upright position is thought not only to help gravity but also to put the woman in the right hormonal balance and reduce the length of labor. Some of the positions mentioned do call for reasonably strong leg muscles. If someone supports you, you can take the strain off your legs.

Pain Relief

You may have gotten the idea that you couldn't possibly get through labor without pain relief. But in fact many women have completely drug-free labors and do not find the pain during natural childbirth unbearable. Indeed, some women actively resist drugs so they can experience childbirth fully and know what this life-changing event feels like.

The other advantage of not using drugs during labor is that neither you nor the baby will be dopey after the birth. Drugs given to the mother reach the baby and affect it too. The baby is more likely to be born fully alert if it has not been given drugs via the mother.

There are several safe alternatives to drugs. Many women find Lamaze breathing techniques or other relaxation methods helpful. You can get some relief from pain by changing position, moving about, being massaged, focusing your concentration, visualization, meditation, self-hypnosis, acupuncture, and acupressure. Some women like dim lighting and gentle music. Some get relief lying in a bath of warm water. It may help to have someone with you to help you relax. Your partner may be very comforting.

Doulas

"The delivery hospital was offering a doula, so we decided that's what we'd do. The doula was very calming. She was quiet and meditative and brought soothing music and aromatherapy oils. The doula knew I had MS, and if it did come to the point where I couldn't push any longer, she knew I might be considered for a cesarean. But I had a natural delivery, and she was a great help."

Doulas can help you get through labor and childbirth calmly. A doula does not have medical qualifications, but she is a woman who has had a child herself and knows what it's like. Traditionally, doulas are calm and reassuring.

Lamaze Techniques

Lamaze training involves special breathing methods that help your body cope with labor pains naturally. You have to go to classes to learn and practice these breathing methods as they cannot be learned from a book. In such classes, you learn to work with your body and trust it. Your partner also learns how to help you during labor.

Transcutaneous Electrical Nerve Stimulation (TENS)

Another drug-free alternative is TENS (transcutaneous electrical nerve stimulation). A small, battery-operated generator is connected by wires to pads that are attached by tape to the skin on either side of the spine. A very low electric current stimulates the nerve endings in the skin and blocks pain signals coming from the uterus. You control the device yourself and vary the strength of the current. It creates a slight buzzing feeling. Some women find it more effective than others. There are no side effects for mother or baby.

Epidural

The most common form of pain relief during labor is epidural anesthesia, which is thought to be safe for MS patients. During the first stage of labor, a fine tube containing an anesthetic drug like the one used by dentists is inserted between two of the spinal vertebrae. This anesthetic numbs nerves carrying sensations from the uterus, cervix, and vagina to the brain. The lower half of your body is also numbed. An epidural is usually effective in deadening the pain of contractions, even though you will still be aware of them. Since MS can itself make you feel numb, epidurals have to be used with extra care.

Once you've had an epidural, it can lead to a cascade of interventions you may not want. You will usually be put on an electronic fetal monitor to check the baby's reactions to the labor. You may also be given medication to counteract the effect of the epidural in lowering blood pressure. And you may need a catheter in your bladder, because sensations are lost from the bladder as well. An epidural will have the effect of slowing down your labor once normal sensations have been numbed. If the epidural has not worn off enough by the end of the second stage of labor, you may not be able to feel when or how to push—the sensations from the pelvic floor are lost. If this happens, the baby may have to be delivered by forceps or vacuum extraction (suction). Forceps deliveries are more common in women who have had an epidural.

Epidural anesthetic does cross the placenta and has an effect on the baby. Some babies seem very jumpy or on edge after an epidural; others are sleepy and difficult to feed for a week or so after delivery.

"They were trying to make me have an epidural. But I didn't fancy the idea of people tampering about with my spine. I'd had three lumbar punctures and didn't want any more needles. I had my first lumbar puncture when I was only eight. I went blind in one eye."

Gas and Air

Gas and air together is a form of inhalation anesthesia. The combination works by changing your perception of pain rather than by anesthetizing you. You breathe in 50 percent nitrous oxide (laughing gas) and 50 percent oxygen through a rubber mask that you control. It can take the edge off the pain, but it cannot deaden it completely. It can make you feel woozy or a little dizzy. Some women feel sick. This mixture is cleared from the baby's system as soon as the baby is born and has started to breathe.

Pethidine or Diamorphine

These are powerful analgesic drugs derived from the same family as morphine. Given by injection into a muscle, they act as muscle relaxants and mood enhancers. These drugs, too, do not take the pain away, but they alter your perception of pain. They can make you feel nauseous; other drugs are sometimes given at the same time to counteract this effect.

These analgesics cross the placenta and may have a marked effect on the baby, both before and after birth. They can affect the baby's breathing and make many babies sleepy; this drowsiness may persist for several days. They can also suppress the baby's sucking reflex. An antidote can be given for the latter symptom.

Steroids During Labor

Patients who have been treated with as little as 10 milligrams of prednisolone daily for more than two weeks during the preceding year may need to be given steroids during labor in order to avoid adrenal insufficiency. In one American center, a typical regimen is 100 milligrams of hydrocortisone injected intramuscularly on admission to the labor room, followed by 100 milligrams every eight hours for twenty-four hours.[3]

Delivery

Induction

In some cases, doctors will induce labor once the cervix has begun to dilate. Contractions tend to be more powerful and can be more painful, but they work to get the baby out.

Forceps and Episiotomy

It is common to have an episiotomy (cutting a wider vaginal opening) and a forceps delivery when an epidural is performed. An episiotomy needs to be stitched and can be quite painful for some time after the birth. And a forceps delivery can sometimes cause complications for both mother and baby. If you tell your doctor you want a natural birth, these interventions and their possible consequences can be avoided.

🖊 *"The doctor did have to use forceps because my muscles weren't strong enough to push the baby out."*

🖊 *"I had a forceps delivery because I couldn't push Siobhan out—I just didn't have the strength anymore. That evening I became incontinent—my bladder started voiding, and I had no control over it. The doctor said the relapse was because I'd had a baby. But even though I did have a relapse from the day she was born, I wouldn't be without my daughter for anything."*

Cesareans

One American study[4] found that the rates of cesareans and instrument-assisted vaginal deliveries are not higher among women with MS. Of eight women with MS studied, only one needed a cesarean section—because her baby was lying in the breech position. A woman with MS should not have a cesarean unless it is essential. It is a major operation. Cesareans are usually given under spinal epidural anesthetic. General anesthesia is also considered safe.

The First Hour after Birth

Immediately after the baby is delivered, he or she should be given to the mother and they should be together for at least the first hour following birth. Ideally, the father should be there too. This is the time for mother and baby to bond emotionally. During this first hour, the baby instinctively finds the mother's nipple and starts to suck. If the mother has had no painkilling drugs during childbirth, the baby is much more alert at this time and begins to explore the senses of sight, sound, touch, taste, and smell.

Leaving the Hospital

Be careful not to ask for discharge from the hospital too soon. You need time to recover from childbirth, and the hospital, where you and your baby are looked after, is a convenient place to begin the process.

Postpartum Depression

If you start getting weepy after the birth of your baby, you may be suffering from postpartum depression. Depression makes you feel that everything in life is awful, and you don't feel up to doing anything. Besides making it very difficult to look after a new baby, depression can also weaken the immune system—which is already compromised in MS. Postpartum depression can be successfully treated with antidepressants. If you do have symptoms, see your doctor.

Having a good relationship with your partner can help protect against postpartum and ordinary depression as well. Measures of "expressed emotion"—which means direct verbal expression by one partner of his or her feelings toward the other—in the partners of pregnant women were found to predict women's psychiatric state after delivery. Women whose partners were positive about them were least likely to become depressed. Those whose partners were uncommunicative about them, neither positive nor critical, were most likely to suffer depression.[5]

Will the Baby Be All Right?

"My baby was beautiful and completely perfect."

Babies are no more likely to be born with defects to mothers with MS than to any other mothers. MS does not have any bad effects in terms of preeclampsia during pregnancy, miscarriages, premature births, stillbirths, or birth defects. A 1994 study of MS and pregnancy concluded, "MS has not been shown to have a deleterious influence on the incidence of toxemia or on the rate of miscarriages, prematurity, infant mortality, and congenital malformations."[6]

9 ✸ Breast-feeding

✺ *"Breast-feeding was so easy and, apart from my baby boy always being attached to a nipple like a limpet, I really enjoyed it. I nursed for more than a year, and it had no effect on my MS at all. But I did lose loads of weight!"*

✺ *"One doctor told me, 'On no account breast-feed,' claiming that every one of his patients who'd done so had become worse."*

There is some disagreement among doctors as to whether breast-feeding is a good idea when you have MS. Their view is influenced by how bad your MS is and what symptoms you have.

In answer to the question "Will I be able to breast-feed?" Dr. Kathy Birk says,

> My answer is generally yes. In the past, neurologists have discouraged nursing, which they thought posed additional demands during a period of increased risk for disease activity. A recent retrospective report found no statistical differences in the risk of timing of postpartum exacerbations between women who nursed and those who did not. Sometimes, however, nursing can be too fatiguing.

The Case for Breast-feeding

Medical opinion agrees that breast milk is best for a baby. Breast milk helps build up defenses in the immune system, and it has all the right ingredients to form a healthy brain. The essential fatty acids found in breast milk are needed for the myelination process of the baby's nervous system, which takes several months. Nursing is also pleasurable and makes the loving bond between mother and baby very strong. It is also very important that the baby get the mother's colostrum right after birth. Colostrum is the substance that comes before the milk starts. It plays a very important part in building up the baby's immunity.

Doctors who are wholeheartedly in favor of nursing point out that it actually requires less effort to breast-feed a baby than to make up bottles. Furthermore, you can nurse a baby in your own bed while still half asleep, whereas you have to get up if you bottle-feed a baby. Looked at this way, nursing can be less tiring. Since breast milk is so good for your baby, it really is worth perservering if you have problems at the beginning. You should not feel guilty if you have to bottle-feed, but it is important to be aware of why breast-feeding is better before switching to bottle-feeding.

The Case against Breast-feeding

Doctors who are against breast-feeding feel that it poses an additional physical burden to women already at risk of a relapse. They say nursing can cause fatigue. In one study, it was found that only 58 percent of MS mothers breast-fed compared with 85 percent of the general population. Half the women who did not breast-feed were advised against it by their doctors.

Where fatigue is a particular concern, or to be prepared in the event of a relapse, some doctors recommend combining breast-feeding with bottle-feeding, using expressed breast milk or, later on, formula milk. This method would allow someone else to feed the baby at night while the mother sleeps. It does not disrupt the milk flow and also gives the father a closer involvement in caring for his baby.

Does Nursing Offer the Baby Protection?

Breast-feeding for at least six months may lower the baby's risk of getting MS later in life. The unique composition of breast milk imparts benefits to the immune system.

There are several reasons why prolonged breast feeding may be associated with a decreased risk of multiple sclerosis. Cow's milk contains lower amounts of unsaturated fatty acids, and a different composition of cortex grey matter has been described in bottle fed infants. This fact could be associated by means of the formation of defective membranes with easier entry of an infective agent across the blood-brain barrier or with accelerated degradation of myelin itself. Human milk might actively influence the immune system of the offspring by different mechanisms, and some features of the immune response among those who have been breast fed for a prolonged period may last for a long time.[1]

Does Breast-feeding Have Any Effect on the Risk of Having a Relapse?

In an American study[2] the exacerbation rate in women who did not breast-feed was 38 percent, compared with 31 percent for those who did. The results do not show much difference. The study found that the average time between childbirth and a relapse for both breast-feeding and non-breast-feeding mothers was three months. Fifty percent of mothers breast-fed, and the average duration of breast-feeding was six months. The study concluded that the hormonal effects of breast-feeding do not lower the risk of exacerbation in the same way that the hormones in pregnancy seem to. When a woman breast-feeds, however, she secretes the hormone pro-lactin. Some doctors think that high secretion of prolactin over a long period of time might be a way to help the immune system recover its pre-pregnancy state.

Healthy Eating

When you're breast-feeding, you are really feeding two people so your nutrition needs to be very good. This means getting enough of all the nutrients you and your baby need. Child-birth and the expulsion of the placenta deplete your body of certain nutrients, which need to be replaced.

- Take zinc and vitamin B_6 to help prevent postpartum depression.

- Take minerals to replace those lost in the placenta and to gain energy and stamina: iron, calcium, mag-nesium, zinc, manganese.

- Take vitamins to increase vitality: B Complex, folic acid, C, A, D, and E.

- Eat adequate amounts of protein.

- Eat plenty. Don't let yourself get hungry or thirsty. Snack during the day on healthy foods, such as wholewheat bread with peanut butter and jam or honey, banana, granola, dried fruits and nuts, fresh fruit, salads.

- Eat only nutritious foods. Give yourself maximum nourishment.

- Drink plenty. Your baby takes between one and two pints of water through your breast milk daily, which you need to replace. Drink as much as six pints of liquid a day.

- Most substances you eat and drink reach your breast milk in varying degrees of concentration. So it is better not to take too much tea, coffee, cola, or other drinks containing additives. Choose healthy drinks like water, herb teas, or fruit juice.

Medications and Breast-feeding

🖎 *"Because I am breast-feeding, my doctor and I are looking at different medical options and what will be compatible. So far, antidepressants are compatible. I would like not to take medication, but I know that may be unavoidable if things stay the same or worsen."*

Betaseron, Avonex, and Copaxone

It is not known whether Betaseron, Avonex, and Copaxone get into human breast milk. The general advice, however, is that they should not be taken while breast-feeding because their effects are not yet well enough understood.[3,4,5] The manufacturers of Betaseron warn that "because of the potential for serious adverse reactions to Betaseron in nursing infants, a decision should be made whether nursing or Betaseron should be discontinued taking into account the importance of the drug to the mother."

🖎 *"I got symptoms about four months after my son's birth. I quit breast-feeding to go on Avonex. Because of dangers associated with the medications I am on I was persuaded to have a tubal ligation so that I would not get pregnant and a baby would not be affected."*

🖐 *"My neurologist wants me to go on Copaxone and stop breast-feeding. He wants me to take the drugs and not have another child. But I want to put my child first. You have to choose between taking the drugs and your child. You are in a very hard place."*

Corticosteroids (Prednisone, Prednisolone, etc.)

If you have a relapse while you are nursing, moderate amounts of prednisone are considered safe for the nursing infant. A few studies have been done that document the presence of prednisone in breast milk after small doses (5 to 10 milligrams). These drugs have shown no adverse effects. Continuous therapy with high doses (10 milligrams or more daily) could affect the infant's adrenal function and should be monitored carefully. Some doctors advise against breast-feeding if you're taking high doses of prednisone or prednisolone because of concern over neonatal bone marrow suppression.

Immunosuppressants (Azathioprine, etc.)

Some specialists in MS advise against breast-feeding when immunosuppressives are necessary, owing to concerns about neonatal bone marrow suppression.

Valium

This drug should be avoided during breast-feeding because it causes lethargy, hypoventilation, and weight loss in the infant. If Valium (diazepam) is thought to be necessary, it is advisable not to breast-feed.

Baclofen

The amounts used are thought to be too small to be harmful to the baby.

Oxybutynin and Propantheline

These medications are not thought to pass into the breast milk.

Vitamin, Mineral, and Other Nutritional Supplements

It's fine to take normal amounts, but do not take excessive doses.

Gentle Therapies

There are gentler alternatives to many of these medications. Holistic therapies also aim to boost the immune system, rather than suppress it. A relaxed state of mind can be achieved by using herbs such as valerian, but check with your doctor to make sure specific herbs are not contraindicated when breast-feeding. Yoga, exercise, meditation, and biofeedback can also reduce anxiety. Spasticity and pain from spasms can be reduced by stretching exercises and using a TENS machine. Bladder problems can be lessened by reflexology. Cranberry juice can sometimes help too.

10 ✸ Getting the Help You Need

❧ *"When I am really tired and in pain there is no backup. I have no support system."*

❧ *"I had a mother's helper from the moment my son was born. I couldn't have managed without her."*

❧ *"I have someone in to do the cleaning and ironing. I can cook, though it's tiring if I stand for too long."*

Babies are unbelievably demanding from the moment they are born, and it is a long time before their need for round-the-clock attention eases off. Even when they are older, children can be exhausting. If you pretend you are just like other mothers (who also get tired), you may be courting disaster.

There are between 250,000 and 350,000 people with MS in North America. About one-fourth of them require help with daily activities or personal care. This burden most often falls on the spouse, who may also have the responsibility of working and looking after the home and children.

"I Was Trying to Do Everything Myself"
✿ Sarah's Story

"I wasn't prepared for the amount of help I would need after the baby was born. I was still in the frame of mind that says you have to live as normal a life as possible. I was trying to do everything myself and was overcome by fatigue. I just had not made allowances that I would need heaps more help than other mothers. I needed protected rest. I needed help with feeding, changing, bathing—everything."

Ideally, you should organize help before the baby is born. If not, do it as soon as you can afterward. You may be able to get help from family, friends, or neighbors. If none of those options is available, you and your partner may have to pay for help yourselves. Money can make all the difference between managing and going under.

🖋 *"When we thought of having a baby, we always planned to have help. We were both working and could afford it. But now that I've gotten worse I've had to give up work completely. My husband doesn't earn enough to support us and pay for help as well. It's a terrible strain on the relationship."*

Asking for Help

🖋 *"I'm too proud to ask for help. Why doesn't anyone offer to help?"*

People sometimes think they ought to be able to cope on their own and feel they have failed if they ask for help. You have to put your baby's well-being and your own health first—which means asking for and getting whatever help you need, even if you must swallow your pride to do so. Some women find this very difficult.

"I'm Not Ready to Admit That I Need Help Yet" ☀ Julie's Story

"I'd have to be immobile before I would take help. I think the stress of letting other people do things for me would be worse than me doing things myself. I don't know these people well enough. I'm not ready to admit that I need help yet. I don't want to have to depend on other people for anything. A workmate of my husband's called and offered to help me, but I told her no because I don't want charity. I'm very stubborn. I walk from one end of a parking lot with my cane because I refuse to ask for a handicapped parking sticker. I walk like I'm eighty, but I don't care. I refuse to give in or give up. No wheelchair, no parking sticker."

Everyone needs help at some time. Give yourself a break—ask for help. There is no need to play the martyr, which can lead to stress, tension, and resentment. If you find it difficult, here are a few tips.

TIPS ON HOW TO ORGANIZE HELP

- Create a team of willing helpers—family, friends, neighbors. You are the team leader. All members have a responsibility to the team. Team members help each other.

- Be specific in what you ask.

- Share out requests for help among your team.

- Don't exaggerate your MS. But be honest and straightforward about it—"My hands are numb now, so I can't cut the bread." Just ask someone to do it.

- Acknowledge that people are helping you. Express your gratitude.

Help from Husbands, Wives, or Partners—
The Effect on Relationships

It's a good idea to talk things through carefully before deciding to have a baby. Once a baby comes along, the partner who does not have MS often has to take on many extra responsibilities that he or she may not have bargained for. This can upset the equilibrium of the partnership. If the wife has MS, the husband may have to do more childcare and housework as well as extra caring for his wife on top of holding down a full-time job. If the husband has MS, the wife may have to become the sole breadwinner on top of her other roles. Getting help organized in advance can ease this strain.

There is a wide variation in how much help the partner with MS gets. Some are blessed with more help than they know what to do with. At the other extreme are those who get no help at all. In some cases, this may be because they feel guilty asking for it. In others, no one suspects they need help because they look so well.

🕊 *"Mark is the most wonderful husband. He gets up early and takes Craig out. They do the shopping together and he does the cooking. He does all this on top of a full-time job. But I reckon if he had to do any more he'd have a nervous breakdown."*

🕊 *"My husband is a great help. He can see when there are days I have done too much and can't walk anymore. He'll watch me walk around the kitchen holding on to the counters, and then he'll say, 'Sit down—you've done enough today.'"*

🖋 *"My husband and I work together. We're a partnership."*

🖋 *"You have to ask yourself, Is your partner going to be able to take on board things in the house? Could he deal with dirty diapers?"*

🖋 *"My husband is not one of life's men who love to care. But I'm sure it's healthier. It's helped me keep responsibility for myself. If I ever needed more personal assistance, he would prefer someone else did it."*

When one of you is disabled, adding a child into the equation can place a greater strain on your relationship. This burden can be eased to some extent by getting practical support. Differences of opinion about the amount of help needed by the person with MS are a common cause of marital conflict. While some spouses do virtually nothing to help, others react the opposite way and do everything, denying the one with MS a sense of ability or independence. Feeling that you are doing more than your fair share can cause deep resentment in a relationship.

"I Was Desperate for Support" ⚙ Leona's Story

"My husband is no help at all. When the baby was born, he disappeared as support. I was desperate for support—emotionally and physically. I had laundry up to the roof, and there were three days' worth of dishes in the kitchen. He expected me to do all the chores—shopping, cooking, cleaning, laundry as well as look after the baby. He's angry at me and the baby for putting so much responsibility on him. The strain is killing him, and he's lost thirty pounds. I feel angry, fed up, and frustrated, and I want a divorce. But I feel tied to him financially, so I can't leave him or move out."

🖋 *"I can't imagine why someone who supposedly loves me so much doesn't want to do things for me and with me."*

🖋 *"All the conflicts in a relationship are accentuated and highlighted when one of you has MS."*

🖋 *"It's a strain on the whole family, whether you realize it or not."*

🖋 *"Having MS has put a lot of strain on the relationship. I have told him many times that I would not hold it against him if he soul-searched and found that he cannot commit himself to give what I need from him emotionally and, as time goes by, physically. I feel that he is trying, but he sees me as a burden and a drain and doesn't feel for me what he seemed to feel before. We are very stressed. I want a trial separation to get some space and perspective, but he doesn't want it."*

🖋 *"Having a child when you've got MS does affect your relationship. My husband is under a great deal of stress and has been seeing a psychologist. It's just the worry and the responsibility."*

It also helps if you lower your standards to realistic levels. Maybe a spot of dust doesn't matter. Maybe it's OK to eat convenience foods. Maybe it's all right if the bathroom doesn't get cleaned quite so often.

🖋 *"My husband never puts any pressure on me about the house or dinner or anything if he knows I'm not feeling the greatest. He always picks up where I leave off. It's hard to say the MS has changed our relationship. Time and circumstance do that. We've been through a lot in eight years and we are closer now than ever."*

Talking Things Over

It's important to have someone you can talk to intimately. It may be that you can share all your concerns and worries with your partner. Or you may need to turn to someone else to spill out what's troubling you. Talking over your anxieties, rather than bottling them up, is very important for your well-being. Whatever problems you have will be less troubling if you can discuss them with another person. Keeping them a secret makes matters much worse.

Help throughout the Years

Typically, MS gets worse over the years. A partner may have to help more and more as time goes on, which can take quite a lot of psychological adjustment on both sides.

🖋 *"Now my husband is having a hard time accepting the reality of the situation and realizing that I need help and that I have not just become a lazy, miserable person. He's a great father, but I don't know how much I could count on him if I had another baby."*

"We Didn't Deal with the Fact That She Had MS" ✿ A Husband's Story

"Leona's MS has had a far greater effect on me than I realized. The spouse is affected, but in a different way. I am definitely affected negatively. Now I suffer a lot of tension-related pain. At the beginning we didn't deal with the fact she had MS. If we didn't deal with it then, how can we deal with it in twenty years' time? It's the scariest thing that has happened to me. It's something you're not prepared for. It's very tough. It's very hard coming to terms with it. It's hard to know the effects it will have on us in the future. I will probably have to take on much more, and I am experiencing pain because of this.

"The timing of the baby wasn't good. Financially, we're not able to cope; we're just scraping by. Leona's not capable of looking after Nicholas twenty-four hours a day. She's quick to point out that she needs help, but she often asks me to do things that she is perfectly capable of doing herself. I get angry about it. Even when she can do it herself, she still asks for help. She's very demanding, and some of her demands are very difficult."

Help from Parents

🖋 *"My mother is seventy-one. When she found out I had MS, she was there for me all the time. I worked as a secretary in the beginning, and she worked also, so the children were taken to a sitter. When I got worse and couldn't work anymore, she cut her hours to help me at home."*

Mothers, and sometimes fathers too, often do a lot to help—even when they may not be in the best of health themselves. If they move in with you, it can create tensions. You may also feel guilty that your mother is doing more than you are. There is always the risk that mothers will treat you like a little girl again, and you may need to be very assertive to resist this inclination. Your mother may also want to raise your children in ways you don't support.

Help from Other Family Members

Extended family members can make a great contribution to raising children and helping with chores.

"My boy has got some great godparents. I've told them that there are some things I can't do and I would like them to do those things for me—running, playing chase, kicking a football. It is very tough on me because I was quite a football player before the MS. I don't know whether I'll be able to bear watching Nick play football with someone else when he's older. It might be too much to take."

When the person with MS doesn't get this help it can add to the stress in his or her life. Some dwell on it, letting it fester inside.

"Not Even My Own Family Cares Enough to Care" ✿ Maria's Story

"My husband has eight brothers and sisters, and I have five. Not once in the two years since my diagnosis did any of them come to visit me, offer to watch my children for an hour, drop off a cooked chicken, or even acknowledge what we were—are —going through. I have pretty much accepted that I am on my own, but when I am in the midst of an attack, it is distressing that there is no one to nurture me. Besides feeling hurt, anger, and loneliness, I feel as if there is something wrong with me that not even my own family cares enough to care."

Help from Friends and Neighbors

Friends and neighbors may not know what help you want unless you tell them. Most people are uninformed about MS symptoms, so don't expect them to know or understand how you feel. You may have to spell it out to them that you tire easily, have bad balance, or are clumsy. If you would prefer them to help with physical things like carrying shopping from the car, rather than looking after your baby—say so! Be nice, but assertive.

You need to be sensitive to their needs too. Friends and neighbors have their own lives to lead; you can't expect them to be at your beck and call all the time. If your demands get too excessive, you could cause resentment. So even if you have helpful friends and neighbors, it is wise to also have other people you could call on in need, such as home health workers, paid help if you can afford it, or volunteers.

"I had one girlfriend who came and spent the day with me several times during my exacerbation. Even though we are no longer close, I will always love her for doing that for me."

"People offered me things I didn't need. They came around and instead of helping or taking the baby so I could rest, I was supposed to entertain them and make coffee."

Help from Your Children

Many parents with MS are very successful parents, managing to raise children who are helpful, caring and loving, and able to do things for themselves from an early age. But it's quite a trick getting the balance right between training your children to be helpful family team members and burdening them with responsibilties that rob them of their rightful childhood.

Few parents want their children to be their own caregivers, but it sometimes happens anyway. Children are sometimes asked to help with not just practical things like shopping and getting meals together, but also more intimate things such as helping a parent get out of bed, go to the toilet, or get dressed. When children have to do all these things in addition to their homework, it can affect their schooling as well as their social life. Some children don't dare go out with friends in case their mother needs them. Taking on the responsibilities of an adult can affect them psychologically. They are losing out on their childhood years and will never be able to get them back.

"We Would Eat, Clean Up, and Begin Homework about Ten" ☼ Steph's Story

"We would eat, clean up, and begin homework about ten. Saturdays and Sundays were workdays too, sometimes at the shop and sometimes housecleaning. My chores were the dishes, cooking when needed, vacuuming, dusting, laundry, cleaning the bathrooms, washing the floors, and trying to pick up a house that seemed to collect clutter better than a trash can. My brother had the outdoor duties—mowing the lawn, taking out the trash.

"What did my father do to help take the pressure off my mom? Well, that's what David and I asked frequently, to no avail. We both hold a lot of resentment for that. He never did some of the things that would have helped Mom more than our housework. He could have paid more attention to what she needed, not what he needed. In the marathon of life, I think circumstances—not a disease—slowed my mom down. But you wait around and watch—she'll finish in the front because her heart is big and her strength is more powerful than she knows."

While children should not be overburdened with housework, they can be trained from an early age to do their fair share of chores and helping out. It is realistic to make your children realize that you cannot do every little thing for them. This is one reason why parents should tell children that they have MS and in what ways it affects the children. Many children are happy to help their mothers with the chores when they see the need. They enjoy being given reasonable responsibilities, especially if you make it like a game.

Children whose mothers have MS often show a high degree of independence as well as a caring and compassionate nature. If you have several children, the older ones can help with the younger ones. Your children will grow up better people if they participate in family life; more caring and loving. Boys especially will benefit. (This applies equally to all families, regardless of MS.)

🖋 *"I ask more of the children, and they're very independent for their age. They fetch and carry things for me. My little boy, who's only two, can climb in and out of his high chair on his own. He has to—I can't haul him in and out of it."*

🖋 *"When Matthew was very little, I showed him how to come down the stairs backward on his own. Friends were amazed that a child so young could do this. But I couldn't have carried him, so he had to."*

🖋 *"The kids pitch in and clear the table and do the dishes. In this family, it's teamwork. My children have grown up with MS, so they know what is expected of them, and I think it makes them better people to be a little responsible. They help me a lot by carrying the laundry down to the basement. They have chores, such as cleaning their rooms, vacuuming, polishing furniture, and so on."*

🖋 *"Steph helps with the laundry and cleaning. Davy helped with meal preparation—he's good. Both the kids did the kitchen cleanup. Their dad didn't do much. He expected them to do all the 'helping.'"*

🖋 *"The boys are very helpful. They understand. They lay the table, load the dishwasher, keep their bedrooms tidy. And I've trained them to change their own bed linen. In the sitting room they are careful not to leave things lying around in case I trip over them. They are always picking things up and putting them away. I think it's a good thing for children to have to do things themselves."*

🖋 *"The kids knew they had to pitch in when I got home. They had to step in and help with the household functions more."*

🖋 *"When I had my third baby, my older children, Bobby and Kerry, were ten and seven. They have been helping me with Michael since he was born. They brought the baby to me when I had to nurse him. Now Michael is five, Kerry gives him a bath and even helps him with his homework."*

TIPS TO MAKE YOUR KIDS WILLING HELPERS

- Treat the family as a team, with different players having different responsibilities.

- When possible, give your kids choices. "This week, would you prefer washing or drying the dishes?"

- Change the chores among your kids so that Bobby doesn't always mow the lawn, for example.

- Have kids share tasks, for example, Bobby and Jane could mow the lawn together. They can decide how and when they are going to do it.

- With kids, make a game out of chores. Who can clean up his or her room the fastest? Can the kids do a better job than dad?

- Remember to praise children for their efforts. "Bobby, you do the dishes better than I do!"

- Free time for play can be the reward for chores completed: Chores first, fun after.

- Structure jobs, for example, the garbage is taken out each night after supper.

- Whining is not allowed.

Domestic Help

🖋 *"Even though I pay people to clean, cook, or look after my children, I am still in control. I'm the one who's running the show."*

🖋 *"I don't want help with the children. I want to do everything with them myself. I don't mind other people doing things like the cleaning. But I don't want anyone else to look after my children. They're my children."*

🖋 *"Now I have full-time help. Someone is here from eight to twelve and two to six. She's a sort of home help/ mother's helper. She gets the younger one off to school, does the housework, and the shopping, runs errands, and makes the children's supper."*

Domestics, Au Pairs, and Nannies

Looking after a home and family involves many energy-sapping chores, like changing bed linen, washing the kitchen floor, ironing, shopping, and food preparation. Many parents with MS prefer to save their energy to be with their children, and have someone else take care of the drudgery, even if they have to pay for it.

To find a willing pair of hands, try putting a small ad in your local paper. You can also find an au pair or nanny through an agency. Au pairs are usually girls under the age of twenty-six from overseas who want to improve their English. They will do a wide range of jobs, including household chores, childcare, and shopping—if you provide a car and they can drive. You pay them "pocket money." The drawbacks are that you need to provide a room for them, and you might feel that having someone living in your home invades your privacy. If you can afford it, you could hire a nanny to help look after your children. Nannies generally will not do any cleaning or general household chores not connected with the children. Because of their specialized training, nannies command far higher wages than au pairs (rates vary—check with a local agency).You may be thankful to have an experienced person, but you may also resent someone else doing what you want to do with your own baby.

🖋 *"I had expected my husband to be able to help me, but he had to go away for his job, and I was all alone. I was so desperate for help that I advertised in the local supermarket so that someone could start the next day. I found a girl who helped me in the house, and she also carried Charlie around for me, since I couldn't even do that. After three months or so, I could walk again with a couple of canes, with the help of a lot of physical therapy. Looking back, it was pretty gruesome, but I was blissfully happy with my baby."*

🖋 *"I am so fortunate to be financially able to afford hired help to babysit, do the laundry, and clean. A majority of women with MS are not so lucky and have to lean much harder on family members, friends, and fellow church members. This requires swallowing your pride and voicing the need for help. Some women have trouble doing that, myself included. These women just wear themselves out trying to do everything themselves and probably put greater strain on their marriages and risk a faster progression of their disease."*

"I am desperate for help, but we are living in poverty. Our debts are terrible. I owe $75,000 toward the costs of my schooling, and $3,500 on credit cards. So we can't afford to pay for help, and I have to do everything myself. It's a nightmare."

Home and Community Waiver Programs

Most state departments of human services offer a home and community waiver program that makes home health aides and other services available. Eligibility requirements and programs differ from state to state but should be investigated with a social worker, the National MS Society, or the county department of human services.

The Medicare Home Health Benefit

If you get Medicare and are homebound, you may be entitled to up to thirty-five hours a week of free skilled nursing on an intermittent basis (fewer than eight hours per day and fewer than seven days per week) as well as home health aide services, and skilled therapy services, provided they are reasonable and necessary. Don't let the complex rules put you off. Skilled nursing includes administration of medications and catheter changes. Skilled therapy covers assessment, therapeutic exercises, gait training, and so on. Home health aide services encompass bathing, feeding, dressing, and toileting.

However, Medicare does *not* cover housekeeping services, such as cleaning or cooking. Your physician must certify the need for care, and a certified home health agency must draw up a plan of care specifying the nature, frequency, and duration of care needed. The benefit is free, except for a 20 percent copayment for durable medical equipment.

11 ✸ Fatigue, Depression, and Other Invisible Symptoms

Some MS symptoms are invisible to other people. You may feel like a wet dishcloth or as if you've gone without sleep for weeks. A hand may be numb, your arms may have pins and needles, your eyesight may be blurred, or your feet may feel like blocks of ice. But to everyone else, you probably look perfectly OK. It is difficult to convince anyone that you need help if you don't have the outward signs of obvious disability, like a wheelchair or a cane.

🐾 *"Fatigue was a major symptom. I should have thought more about how I was going to manage."*

🐾 *"My husband thought that because I was at home all day and not out at work I should be able to take care of the baby and the apartment. He just doesn't understand the fatigue."*

🐾 *"I got totally exhausted within weeks. The MS continued to get worse."*

🐾 *"My baby wanted feeding all the time. I was doing the housework, the cooking, and the shopping. And I never got a complete night's sleep for a long time."*

🐾 *"Sometimes I believe my husband's family thinks that if the MS is not visible and we don't talk about it, then it doesn't exist. It's pretty odd that we don't verbalize anything. If I say I'm tired to my mother-in-law, she'll say,*

'Oh, I've been a little tired lately too. Guess it's the weather.'"

🖋 *"I've been refused disability payments because my neurologist says I'm OK to work. But the fatigue is so bad that I can't even carry the baby. People around me say, 'Just deal with it!' It doesn't help that I look so well! Being fatigued doesn't tally with looking attractive and healthy. My husband, Yusuf, is finding it a terrible strain. But if he's like this now, when I still look attractive, what will he be like if I get worse and become more disabled?"*

Fatigue

For many people, fatigue is the worst of all the invisible symptoms of MS because you have no energy to do even the simplest of tasks. It makes looking after a child much more difficult. Even when you say you're tired, other people may look at you and think you look perfectly all right. This makes it particularly difficult for wives who are expected by their husbands to do stereotypically female tasks such as housework, cooking, and shopping—as well as looking after the baby and looking good too.

It's not unusual for people to brand you as lazy or a slob if you don't accomplish everything. And if you complain, they may think you're neurotic. Indeed, you may feel guilty about it yourself and think that you really are a lazy and neurotic slob. You must explain to those around you—husband, mother-in-law, neighbors, or whoever—that the fatigue is real and that if you overdo it you could make yourself worse. In some relationships, this may take a lot of sorting out and there could be conflict. But it is better to try to straighten things out than to let matters fester, causing resentment and distance. On the other hand, there may be things that you can do at times when your fatigue isn't too bad. Doing all that you realistically can helps you perceive yourself as an active, useful person, rather than someone who is ill and lazy.

"People Think I'm Lazy, But I'm Not" ✿ Avril's Story

"One of the problems is that I look so well that people can't understand there's anything wrong. I don't get much support from my family. When I say I can't do things, my mother says, 'Why don't you just try?' It makes me so angry because people think I'm lazy, but I'm not.

"By the end of the day, all I want to do is flake out and do nothing. But I can't. I always have to push myself on and drag myself around—preparing a meal, giving her a bath, reading her a story, and putting her to bed. My daughter knows there's something wrong with her mom, but I think she's too young to understand exactly what it is. I don't know how to handle telling her."

Fatigue in MS is not like normal fatigue, from which you can recover quite quickly with a good rest. It is chronic fatigue, where everything seems to be an effort. You feel like a radio with run-down batteries. MS fatigue is not just about tired muscles. Fatigue stems from the effect of the disease on the nerves that go to the muscles, and also on the sensory nerves. Fatigue in MS may also be caused by lack of oxygen to the muscles from poor circulation or shallow breathing. The most common triggers of fatigue are: overexertion, overdoing it, lack of sleep and rest, stress, heat, humidity, hot baths, hunger, food allergies, and nutritional deficiencies.

There are several potentially effective ways to combat fatigue:

- Get plenty of rest and a good night's sleep.

- Take a nap during the day.

- Exercise enough to get oxgyen traveling through your body.

- Do yoga or deep breathing exercises.

- Eat little and often; never skip breakfast.

- Avoid stress.

- Keep cool; turn up the air conditioning, suck on ice cubes, sit next to a fan, or lie back in a pool of tepid water.

- Give up eating foods to which you are allergic.

- Try food combining (also known as "The Hay Method") in which you don't mix proteins and carbohydrates at the same meal.

- Drink plenty of water.

- Lose weight if you're overweight.

One hypothesis concerning fatigue in MS is that the food that you eat is not being absorbed properly by the gut. This malabsorption may be due to candidiasis, a yeast infection that can be treated by a nutritionally oriented doctor (see chapter 4). Cut back on sweet, sugary foods, refined carbohydrates, fermented foods, and yeast.

Depression

Depression is common in MS. If you have just had a baby, you are also at risk of postpartum depression. But don't worry too much—you are more likely to feel joy and euphoria after you've had a baby.

🖋 *"I'm so in love with my baby, I'm on a permanent high!"*

The telltale signs of depression are profound sadness, loss of interest in everyday activities, changes in appetite and sleep patterns, feelings of worthlessness and/or guilt, lassitude, and thoughts of death or suicide. A major depressive episode will sap your ability to function, and you may withdraw from daily life and social interactions. If you have any of these symptoms, see your doctor. You don't have to suffer in silence.

Major depressive illness is more common in MS patients than in the population in general and in other disability groups. About half the people who have MS will experience a full-blown, major episode of depression at some time. It is more likely to happen during an exacerbation. Fatigue makes depression worse; try to rest, get the sleep you need, and ask others for help. Depression can be successfully treated with medications alone or in combination with psychotherapy, which should be done one-to-one with a psychiatrist, psychologist, or social worker. Treatment can shorten the episode and prevent or delay future episodes.

The medications that work best for depression in MS are the selective serotonin re-uptake inhibitors (SSRIs) such as Prozac, Zoloft, Paxil, and Effexor. These should be used with caution during breast-feeding, and only if there is a compelling need. They are thought to be safe, but this depends on dose, the age of the infant, and the timing of the dosage. Consult a physician who knows about drugs during breast-feeding.

St. John's wort is a natural alternative to the pharmaceutical antidepressants. However, orthodox physicians are not convinced of its effectiveness or safety. Until the efficacy of St. John's wort for the treatment of major depressive disorder is firmly established and its reproductive safety is evaluated more thoroughly, the tricyclic antidepressants and fluoxetine (Prozac) appear to be safer alternatives.[1]

Postpartum depression is sometimes caused by a hormonal imbalance, and in some cases can be treated with progesterone.

Women who take vitamin B_6 and zinc after giving birth are less likely to experience postpartum depression.

"The Smallest Task Is Overwhelming"
✪ Emily's Story

"I have never been so depressed in all my life. Suddenly the smallest task is overwhelming. I feel pathetic and empty. Mostly I have felt out of control. I say to myself, 'Why can't I just overcome this thing?' My husband has come home from work early because of it.

"I do worry for my children, especially the oldest—about what he is missing out on because I can't play with him, that I'm so angry and depressed, or that I can't pick him up the way I used to. He will often ask me, 'You not feeling well, Mommy?' When my husband gets home, he says, 'Mommy weak, Daddy.' He deserves better."

🖋 *"Some days I'm very down, and if I didn't have a child there have been times when I might have thought of end-*

ing it all. But I only have to think of her, and I keep going. She is my purpose in life. Having a child gives me the will to go on."

Mood

When you are fatigued, you can take it out on your children with irrational bouts of bad temper. If you are aware that this can happen, you can try to prevent it, nip it in the bud, or ask someone else to look after the children while you rest and recover your equilibrium. If you feel stress getting to you, take time out to be on your own and relax. Humor is always a good way to defuse tension—try making a joke of things instead of getting steamed up. You can control your moods more easily than you may realize. You can make a decision to be less negative and gloomy. People with MS can often give themselves a hard time, blaming themselves for the slightest silly little thing that goes wrong. Try not to be too perfectionist, and don't kick yourself too much when you foul up. We're all human.

🖋 *"When I am really tired and they are just being the children that they are, I sometimes lose my temper with them. I always apologize and reinforce that I need them to behave when I am sick. But I see the damage I am doing. I try so hard to hang on, hang on, but I feel I am breaking physically and in every other way that a person can break."*

🖋 *"The worst aspect of the MS with children is the times it affects my mood. I love my boys so much, and I want to give them everything they need emotionally. But sometimes I am depleted, and then my husband has to double up."*

Cognitive Problems and MS

🐾 *"I'm sure I've lost at least thirty-two IQ points since getting MS."*

Although it is not often openly talked about, cognitive problems can develop in MS. Your brain processes will not work 100 percent. These problems can affect memory, attention, concentration, and the ability to find the right words. Information processing is slowed down, and reasoning, problem solving, and judgment are impaired. Visual and spatial abilities are also affected. All these impairments have an impact on being a parent. Other people—even family members who don't fully understand what is happening in MS—may begin to think of you as forgetful, unreliable, insensitive, lazy, selfish, or just plain stupid. Teenagers may think you are "dumb" and tell you so. This can lead to anger, confusion, and strain in the family, which can create a climate of tension, anxiety, and sadness in the home. The best solution is to discuss what is happening and why and to come up with ways to solve some of the problems caused by cognitive changes. For example, if poor memory is a problem, writing things down can help.

12 ❀ Having More Children

Many mothers with MS have several children—some as many as five. Some have no qualms about having more children, regardless of MS. Others can feel a great deal of conflict. They have to weigh the longing for another baby against the risk of possibly getting worse and worries about whether they could cope. In addition, they may face opposition from family members and physicians. If a couple decides against having more children, they can sometimes feel sad about never having the son or daugher they wanted, or a sibling for their only child.

❧ *"I now want another baby, and my mother is having a cow. She says, 'What if this?' and 'What if that?'"*

❧ *"Sometimes we get all broody, and we'd like to have another child. But I seem so stable and happy at the moment we think having another one might upset the applecart."*

❧ *"We did want a third child. But I was getting fatigued all the time, and we thought, 'Can we cope?' The doctors said we shouldn't. If I didn't have MS I would certainly have had more children. But we began to say, 'What if . . . ?'"*

❧ *"I would like to have had a daughter as well as a son. But when he was about one I said to myself, 'No, this is too much like hard work!'"*

🎋 "When my little boy was two years old, I had a relapse on holiday and suddenly couldn't walk. I felt we couldn't cope with another baby."

🎋 "I would love to have had another child, but it wouldn't have been fair on Siobhan. My health might have been jeopardized."

🎋 "It wouldn't have been fair to my husband to look after three of us. Two he could manage—but not three!"

"I Ache to Have Another" ✹ Maria's Story

"I really was planning on having another. You know, go for the girl or have a round number of three sons. Now, as much as I ache to have another, I feel it would be crazy. I can't part with any of my baby things, just in case. I almost wish I would have an 'accident' so that I didn't have to make that decision. I am having a hard time adjusting. I was a very active, forward-moving graphics designer and seriously dedicated to being a wife and mother. Now I can't keep up with my life as it is. Logically, I think having another would be selfish, but my heart feels that all the love I, my husband, and two big brothers have to give would make up for my inability to be a very physical mother."

Two medical studies have found that there was no connection among the number of children, timing of pregnancies, and long-term disability.[1] One population-based study in Canada published these conclusions: "We found no differences in the long-term disability of women with no pregnancies, one pregnancy, or two or more pregnancies. . . .

Pregnancy per se or number of pregnancies has no effect on subsequent disability."[2]

Despite these findings, it is still quite common for mothers with MS to be advised by their doctors not to have a second or third child. In a study carried out in England,[3] three mothers found the medical arguments persuasive and accepted this advice. Two of the three decided to terminate their pregnancies. One woman's consultant told her, "You got away with two. Don't tempt fate by having a third." Two women had gone ahead with unplanned third pregnancies because they did not want terminations, for religious or other reasons. Both felt they had incurred the anger of health professionals for this choice.

🖋 *"My [male] doctor strongly advised termination of my present pregnancy. He thinks that a single parent of two with multiple sclerosis cannot possibly cope with three children."[4]*

🖋 *"When I wanted to have a third child, my neurologist did not yell at me, but he told me that it would be hard and he hoped I had a supportive husband and family. I had both."*

🖋 *"The doctor said, 'Now that you have a baby, we want you to go on medication. If you want to have more children, you will have to go off Copaxone for six months and go through two cycles of menstruation.' He said we don't know whether this drug has any harmful effects on a fetus or whether it affects a woman's eggs. There just isn't the research. It's very scary."*

Siblings

In some ways having two or more children eases the burden for the mother once they are past babyhood, because, if they are near enough in age, they play (and fight!) with each other rather than endlessly demanding their mother's time, attention, and energy.

🪶 *"The biggest area that brings me sadness is that of siblings for my son. He desperately wants them, but I am fearful it will not be."*

🪶 *"Nobody shares your childhood with you like a sibling does. When you're grown up it goes on being important."*

🪶 *"My son begged me for a little sister. But I told him I couldn't. Now I regret it. It would have been much easier if there had been two of them, since they could have played with each other instead of him always wanting my total attention."*

🪶 *"I wanted to have the two children as close together as possible so they could be playmates. Now the boys always do things together, and I have quite an easy time of it."*

🪶 *"The advantage of having three children is that they have each other. They can help each other out and really enjoy each other's company. On the other hand, they also fight like crazy sometimes. I think it would have been easier on me, both physically and emotionally, to have just one or two, but I would not change a thing. When I watch them give each other hugs before bed, it warms my heart."*

Abortion (also see "Abortion" in chapter 3)

If you get pregnant and feel you could not cope with another baby, a termination may be the option you choose. Make sure you're not being pressured into it. And also remember that there are risks involved in having a termination: you have the same chance of having a relapse as if you had a full-term baby. Think this over carefully, because acting too quickly and then regretting your decision can have psychological effects for a long time.

🖋 *"My OB/GYN even had the nerve to ask me if I wanted to continue with the pregnancy. I told her that God gave me MS and God gave me this baby and everything is for a reason. I would not even think about terminating my pregnancy."*

🖋 *"When I found I was pregnant with my third child I seriously considered having an abortion. It was difficult enough looking after my two boys without another one on top. But then I talked it over with my husband and we decided to go ahead. Now I have the most beautiful baby girl in the whole world and am so happy."*

Sterilization

🖋 *"My doctor asked me if I would like a sterilization. I was only twenty-six and hardly affected by MS. I was so dumbfounded that I just stood there. How could this man even suggest such a thing? I was shocked and horrified. Of course I said no. I had a baby a few years afterward."*

"He Said He Thought It Was Better for Me if I Didn't Have Any More Children" ✿ Beverley's Story

"When I was seven months pregnant with my second child and very well, a doctor offered me a sterilization. He said he thought it was better for me if I didn't have any more children. I was livid. I said, 'No way!' They were going to sterilize me at the same time as my second baby was being born. He obviously thought I wouldn't be able to manage with more than two children. . . . What made me so angry was that he expected me to say yes."

One medical study concluded, "Frequent expressions of regret after sterilization suggests that reversible methods of contraception might be preferable."[5]

13 ☀ Adoption

Until quite recently, doctors sometimes recommended that a woman with MS adopt a child rather than have a baby of her own—they feared a relapse following childbirth. Although it is true that having a baby can make MS worse, it is probably just as tiring looking after an adopted child. In any case, women with MS who have children do rather better in the long run than childless women. It is also worth considering the emotional issues involved in adopting a child. Children adopted from orphanages can sometimes suffer from emotional damage that cannot be remedied by being with a loving family. Following the publicity of the "Baby M" case in 1985, it was widely believed that women with MS put their health at risk if they have their own babies. This case also shows that going through the adoption process can be very stressful.

On the other side of the coin, it can also happen that a woman with MS feels she cannot cope with bringing up a child and thinks about giving up her own child for adoption.

🖋 *"I seriously considered giving up the baby. I didn't want him not to have a good life. I felt I couldn't give him all the things I have inside me—the love, the knowledge, the education."*

🖋 *"If it's dangerous for her to have another child, I'd like to adopt. I don't want to make her life more difficult if a baby's going to make it worse."*

🪶 *"We have discussed having a family and adopting an older child. We both are extremely concerned with overpopulation and decided years ago that adoption would be the only way we would ever have a family."*

🪶 *"I'm not sure I could adopt. I would rather go through with the dangers of having a relapse and have my own child."*

The "Baby M. Case"

Dr. Elizabeth Stern was a pediatrician with a mild case of MS. She was advised that pregnancy could worsen her disease and make her work difficult, if not impossible. Her career was very important to her, and she did not want to jeopardize it. For this reason, Dr. Stern and her husband, William, made a contract in 1985 with Mary Beth Whitehead in which Mrs. Whitehead would be a surrogate mother. She was to be artificially inseminated by Mr. Stern's sperm. This meant that Mrs. Whitehead would be the child's biological mother—not Dr. Elizabeth Stern. Mrs. Whitehead agreed to give the child to the Sterns after giving birth. She also agreed to give up her parental rights in return for a payment from the Sterns of ten thousand dollars plus her medical bills.

But when Mary Beth Whitehead gave birth to a baby girl, she changed her mind and refused to give the child to the Sterns. The Sterns took legal action to gain custody of the child and deprive Mrs. Whitehead of all parental rights, including the right to see her child. The case became known as the "Baby M. Case" because the Sterns named the baby Melissa.

The case was hotly contested and raised many issues. In the end, the New Jersey State Supreme Court decided that the contract was not valid. The payment of money to a surrogate mother was "child selling" and therefore illegal; surrogacy was potentially demeaning to women because surrogacy made people think of them as "walking wombs." Last, Mary Beth Whitehead was given parental rights to Baby M. As both Mr. Stern and Mrs. Whitehead had parental rights to Baby M., the court had to decide which parent was best fit to have custody of her and which arrangement would be in the best interests of the child.

This is where multiple sclerosis played a part. MS had been the main reason why the Sterns had approached a surrogate mother—they feared having a baby of her own would make Dr. Stern's MS worse. Experts called by Mrs. Whitehead's lawyers disputed the risk of pregnancy to Dr. Stern, however, and portrayed her as placing her career before a child.

A court order gave Mr. Stern temporary custody of Baby M. When this happened, Mrs. Whitehead fled with the baby, her husband, and her other two children. A few months later, during a phone conversation with Mr. Stern, Mrs. Whitehead was taped as saying: "I'd rather see me and her dead before you get her." This tape, together with other factors, set the odds against Mary Beth Whitehead. The court made a unanimous decision to award custody to Mr. Stern. A separate hearing determined how often Mrs. Whitehead could visit Baby M. Because Mrs. Whitehead retained parental rights, Dr. Elizabeth Stern was not allowed to adopt "Baby M."

There are cases of adoption where the man has MS. The couple can decide to adopt because either the husband or wife has fertility problems, or because there is a genetic risk. One father said: "We didn't want to pass along our genes to a child. I have MS, my dad has Parkinson's, and breast cancer runs in my wife's family."

"Life with Daddy in the Slow Lane"
✿ Gordon's Story

"Were we crazy to adopt a baby from Paraguay in 1994? Thanks to MS, my mobility and eyesight are poor. Nonetheless, Eli knows he is a very special part of our family. MS posed no problems adopting in Paraguay. At the time, adoption was one of Paraguay's biggest industries. The country loves the U.S. dollar. Many single women adopt there. Adopting in Paraguay is no hassle at all—just a big expense. It came to about thirty thousand dollars, but worth every penny.

"Giggle-box Eli had nothing to adjust to growing up with a daddy with 'weak legs.' That's because life with Daddy in the slow lane was normal, routine. What's more, since I have an electric scooter, Eli and I experience so much together on the road. We traveled to Disney World, the world's most accessible environment, for a week. At home we explore huge shopping malls and enjoy swimming pools near our home. Eli's big question? 'Why don't other daddies drive a scooter?'

"Half the time Eli is *my* guardian angel, taking care of *me*. He delivers my cane when I need it, transports my lunch to our den from the kitchen, and gives me terrific directions in the car when I get lost. Even at the Disney World Resort in Florida, he had a better sense of direction than I did when he was copilot on my scooter, trying to find our hotel room. Like any child, Eli has cranky days, cries, gets sick, and attempts activities that are off limits. But all told my wife and I couldn't have created a more loving, caring, sensitive son. Let's hope he doesn't lose these characteristics. I know he will always help me retain an upbeat spirit, MS and all."*

---

*Thanks to Gordon Chesy from Hartsdale, New York, and his local MS Society chapter.

14 ☀ Single Mothers

🖋 *"I feel pretty scared about raising a child on my own—
confident in my commitment but scared of the day-to-day
reality and especially the long-term effects."*

Few women with MS set out to become single mothers. But
some end up that way, either through unplanned pregnancies,
divorce, separation, or because they have parted from their
boyfriends. Others simply do not want to get married. If the
father is still in the picture, the child has the benefit of both a
mother and a father even if he or she lives mainly with one
parent.

If there is no father around, a single woman only has to
think about herself and her child. In some ways this is easier,
but she may have to do everything on her own. Once again,
money and social support make a big difference. Some mothers with MS who have become single are working in well-paid
jobs and can afford high-class childcare and home household
help. Those without spare cash to pay for help can find being
a single mother very tough.

🖋 *"My nanny is wonderful—smart, sweet, fun, and with a
good knowledge of the types of child-rearing I prefer. She
speaks great English, and she drives! This opens whole new
worlds for Matthew in terms of even more park possibili-
ties, play dates—anything. It gives me great peace of mind
that he has a full, fun, and enriching daily existence."*

Even today, though, being a single mother can sometimes
be a social stigma and you may not get support from parents
or other family members who may disapprove of what you
have done.

"Being a Single Mother with MS Is a Real Struggle" ☀ Avril's Story

"I became pregnant when I was abroad and didn't even realize it until I was several months gone. By then it was too late to have an abortion. The man was just a brief fling and didn't even know about it. I had no idea when I was due and had no prenatal care at all. The baby was born in the Emergency Room. My parents wouldn't help because I was having an illegitimate child. A social worker came to the hospital with all the papers for an adoption. She expected me to sign over my daughter for adoption without any fuss. But when I held my daughter and looked at her beautiful face, I knew I couldn't give her up and refused permission.

"At that time I hadn't been diagnosed with MS, even though I'd had symptoms before she was born, which they said was encephalitis. But soon after the birth I was dragging a foot and had problems with my vision and really bad fatigue. I told my doctor I wasn't well, but no one's going to offer you any help unless you have a clear-cut diagnosis. It was very hard managing on my own. It went on like that until my daughter was four, when at last I got a diagnosis of MS. Daily life is hard. I can manage only small amounts of shopping since I find carrying heavy bags very difficult. Not everyone has been helpful. Being a single mother with MS is a real struggle."

The positive side of being a single mother is that a baby can give you joy and a sense of fulfilment you otherwise may not have had.

"It's the Right Decision for Me—One That's Made Me the Happiest I've Been in Quite a While"
☼ Belinda's Story

"Unfortunately, my partner and I split up before the pregnancy was detected. I was very depressed and thought the only thing to do would be to have a termination as I was taking medication that can cause birth defects. I also thought that being single and having MS, I wouldn't be able to cope and that it would be cruel to bring up a child with this sort of life. However, I decided not to terminate the pregnancy. Of course, I still worry, but I know it's the right decision for me— one that's made me the happiest I've been in quite a while."

If your child has access to his or her father, this can sometimes make life easier for you as it gives you a break. You can be on your own and do whatever you want to do. Far from missing their children, some women find they enjoy a regular breather, as long as it's not too long.

"It Gives Me Much More Freedom" ☼ Naomi's Story

"My son lives half the time with his father and half the time with me. I don't have the energy any longer to look after him all the time, anyway. When he's with his dad he can do energetic things I can't do, such as skiing. And I can have a total break from cooking, washing clothes, and shopping. I can get up late in the morning, go to the beauty shop when I want to, have a rest, or go to bed whenever I feel like it. It gives me much more freedom. My son seems OK with the arrangement. Anyway, a lot of his friends live in two separate homes —sometimes with their mom and sometimes with their dad. These days it's common."

15 ❊ Practical Tips on Looking after a Child

Doing everyday things that other people take for granted without a second thought can be daunting when you have MS. Carrying a baby and all its paraphernalia up and down steps, going shopping, and even changing diapers can be difficult when your balance is bad, fatigue is overwhelming you, and you're clumsy. When you see other "normal" mothers doing things so easily, you can start feeling inadequate and sorry for yourself. But this can only lead to gloom. Try not to compare yourself. You can be sure your baby loves you, even if you do sit down in the park rather than run around. Just do what you can and enjoy your child.

🌾 "I fear I won't be able to do what normal people do with young children. I get jealous of people running in the park."

🌾 "I can't always do what other mothers do. I can't go on school trips, since I can't walk distances."

🌾 "I would like to go out more with her, but I can't drive. We're very limited to where we can go in the wheelchair— where we live is so hilly."

🌾 "I can't do things spontaneously. Every outing is a production; it needs so much organization."

🌾 "My walking's not bad enough for a wheelchair but not good enough for trudging across theme parks. My son hates me dragging along behind him so slowly. He some-

times says, 'I wish you weren't disabled, Mommy.' I say, 'So do I.'"

🖎 *"Somebody once told me, 'If you're disabled, they won't run off.' It's not true."*

Not all problems can be solved with a quick fix. With more help, better access, and the right equipment, however, some of them can be tackled and overcome. There will probably be things you cannot do with your children, and other people will have to do them for you. But that doesn't make you any less of a parent.

Hints and Tips from Other Mothers

The following tips on how to make life easier with a baby or young child come from other mothers who have MS.

- Learn to ask for help and accept the offers.

- Rest when you feel the need.

- Have everything close at hand. One mother says: "For the baby I have all the supplies I will need by my chair—diapers, wipes, changing pad, garbage bag. She has a little cradle I can put her in by the chair as well."

- Have changing equipment and other paraphernalia downstairs as well as upstairs.

- Have the baby sleep next to your bed or in your bed with you, so you don't have to get up at night.

- The more labor-saving devices you have, the less work and fatigue for you.

- Save your energy so that you have enough energy left to play with your children.

- Plan things. If you are going on an outing, plan the route and all the details before you leave. It will save you from getting frazzled on the journey.

- You may not be able to run after a toddler who's into everything, so make sure your home is safe. Put safety gates at tops and bottoms of stairs and to block exits, get a kettle guard and a stove guard, and put breakable ornaments out of reach.

- Think of all the things you *can* do, rather than the things you can't.

- Stay cool—air conditioning or a good fan. It helps prevent fatigue.

- Train your children to respect your needs.

"It's a Commitment to a Life" ✲ Maria's Story

"I think any new mother should know what she is getting herself into. It's not playing house. If she makes a decision to have a child, she has to realize that it's a commitment to a life. She has to think about creative ways of handling her role as a mom. She is not going to be able to do all the things that other mothers do. You have to find your own way to handle being involved in your child's life—cub scouts, school parties, baseball, and so forth."

🖋 *"It was so important to rest that I trained my five-year-old not to bother me unless he saw blood or fire. We still joke about that to this day."*

Make Life Easy for Yourself

Wheelchairs, Scooters, and Other Aids and Equipment

There are so many aids and pieces of equipment on the market that can make life easier (see appendix A for a database of adaptive equipment), but you need to have the right attitude toward them. View them simply as useful things. Like cars, wheelchairs get you places. Whatever aids you choose, see them as nothing more than that—aids. They are not badges that say "this person is disabled, poor thing." Those attitudes are no longer valid in today's society.

- Use a wheelchair or electric scooter when you need to. It's easier to get around and saves on legs and energy. Don't worry about what other people think. Wheelchairs can also be used in games with the children.

- Take a lightweight portable chair with you when you go out so you can sit down at any time.

- Use a cart instead of carrying things on a tray.

- If stairs are a problem, install a stairlift.

- If you get tired standing in the kitchen while preparing food, get a "perching stool."

- If you lose your balance easily, get a sturdy walker.

- As signs of MS aren't always obvious, it can help to carry a cane so that other people don't question whether or not you have a disability.

- Get a "handicapped" parking sticker so you can park in "handicapped only" parking spaces.

- If talking or writing is a problem, get a computer with voice-recognition software and an internet connection.

Many mothers and fathers with MS feel left out of activities. But with the help of wheelchairs, electric scooters, and other adapted equipment, it is possible to join in much more than you may have thought. These days, having a handicap is no bar to such things as skiing, sailing, or visiting places, for example. It's easy to use MS as an excuse for not engaging in many activities. You'll get more fun and pleasure out of life, and enjoy more things with your children, if you find ways to do the things you want to do.

"I know I do more than some mothers who don't have MS. I guess that's because I hate being told I can't do something. I go to Little League baseball games, take my daughter to dance class, do all my own cooking and housecleaning. I even work in the garden."

"When my daughter wants to go to the mall, I pack up my electric scooter, and off we go. When my son has a Little League baseball game, I bring my cane, a chair, and my video camera, and off I go. Nothing stops me from having a good time."

"The boys used to think it was great fun that I had to sit down on a chair to play soccer with them. They thought it was great because no other mom played soccer in a chair."

🖋 *"The bonus of a wheelchair is that you can have them on your knee and whizz about. They love that. Walking would be so much harder."*

🖋 *"I have an electric wheelchair and can go almost anywhere. It's marvelous."*

🖋 *"When MS joined the family, I could still enjoy the Washington Fair in a wheelchair. I think the kids felt bad, different, and mad at first, but it meant we could enjoy the same thing we had done for years."*

🖋 *"I hate being a wheelchair user. You are pushed about. It's a very passive existence. But at the same time, what a difference it's made to me having a wheelchair with a child on my lap."*

🖋 *"You can move very fast in this wheelchair. When he was a toddler and he got up to some mischief, I'd whizz over to him and take him by surprise."*

🖋 *"I spend the entire summer in the pool. It's the only place I feel comfortable. If I stay out in the sun, my body shuts down; I can't stand on my legs. But once I was in the pool, I could walk out half an hour later. It's amazing what the heat can do."*

Live Somewhere Accessible

Babies and young children need a lot of stuff that has to be carried from your home to the car and back again—carseats, diapers, changing bag, toys, bottles, and so on. So choose a place to live where it's not going to be a daily hassle.

🖋 *"Before the baby was born, we moved to an apartment three flights up at the top of a house. It's thirty-six steps up, and thirty-six steps down. I have to keep on stopping on the stairs. It's a nightmare getting the baby's stuff up and down the stairs."*

Trying to Be like Other Parents

🖋 *"When I can barely get to a baseball game and all of the healthy mothers are bouncing around, I feel like I am not being the mother they want me to be. Both of my boys are very sensitive to me, and I know they see me trying to do for them and be with them. But I always see what I can't do."*

🖋 *"When Nick wants to go out, I have to get the electric scooter out of the garage, and it's all a bit of a palaver. With any ordinary father, he'd be able to just go out for a walk."*

It's unreasonable to be too hard on yourself. What's important is that you are doing your best. It's not helpful to compare yourself with other people. Some parents feel inadequate because of the way they look or the things they can't do, but there is no need to feel this way. Your children love you the way you are.

Don't be a perfectionist or make ridiculous demands on yourself as a parent. No parent is perfect. There is no set way of being a good parent. All parents are better at doing some things than others—that's normal. Concentrate on what you *can* do rather than moan about what you *can't* do. It's much more important to relate to your children than to play ball with them. Talk to your children. Listen to what they say. Love them.

"I Am There for Them Emotionally"
✸ Jeanne's Story

"I get frustrated at times when I am sitting on vacation while my husband and the kids are all off climbing and biking or whatever. But I am there for them emotionally, which I think is much more important in the definition of motherhood than being able to do physical things, such as ski or go hiking with them. I have seldom missed any big moments in their lives—dance recitals, sports, school programs—so that has been great!"

How to Handle People Who Don't Understand

Even today, some people are hostile to the idea of disabled women having children at all and think they must make bad parents because they can't look after their children like "normal" mothers. The idea that women with MS are unfit mothers unfortunately still holds with some people, but it seems to be on the wane. What other people say about you doesn't make it so. You don't have to listen to them. You can confront them, challenge them, joke about it, educate them, or be rude. Other people have their opinions and attitudes. You can only upset yourself by paying attention to them. Don't worry yourself about it—it's not worth the effort.

"There Was an Assumption That Rachel Couldn't Have Had Her Own Child" ✿ Mark's Story

"When we go out, we sometimes get weird looks if Rachel's in a wheelchair. It's incredible, a real ingrained attitude. It makes no difference how old they are. The other week we went into a shop with Craig, and what we wanted to buy was upstairs. Craig made for the stairs, but, of course, Rachel couldn't get up them because of the wheelchair, and there was no elevator. One woman said, 'You shouldn't have a child if you can't get upstairs.'

"One or two people have said, 'You shouldn't have been so irresponsible as to have children.' The other week we were shopping, and we saw someone we knew. She looked at Craig and said, 'Where did you get that child from?'—as if we'd borrowed him or something. There was an assumption that Rachel couldn't have had her own child because she was in a wheelchair. If you're disabled, some people just expect you to sit at home all day long and be looked after."

"I Got a Letter Saying a Woman with MS Couldn't Be a Proper Mother" ✿ Anthea's Story

"My ex-husband and I had the most horrendous custody battle over my son. The stress was unbelievable. I physically fell to pieces, and five months later I was told I had MS. While I was in the hospital after the diagnosis, I got a letter from my husband's lawyer saying that a woman with MS couldn't be a proper mother. He demanded a full report from the neurologist to use against me in the divorce court.

"Luckily, I had the most wonderful neurologist. As chance would have it, his own mother had MS, and he said he couldn't

see any reason why I couldn't be a good mother. The judge
gave me custody of the child."

Getting Support from Other Mothers with MS

🌾 *"I was keen to meet other mothers with multiple sclerosis, and it took a lot of work to find them. It is only recently
that I've met other disabled mothers who've become good
friends."*

You may feel the need to meet other parents who have been
through or are going through experiences similar to yours.
You are certainly not the only one. Finding other mothers
with MS means you can share concerns, give mutual support,
and not feel isolated. You can find other parents with MS
through MS Society chapters or via the Internet (see appendix A).

16 ☀ Older Children

☛ *"It definitely gets easier as they grow older. They are more helpful, and they can understand when you need their help."*

☛ *"My boy is eleven now and he still wants me to do everything and go everywhere with him. I long for the day when he's old enough to go off on his own. I know it's awful to wish away his childhood, but at least it would give me a breather, and I'd be able to sit down and put my feet up now and then."*

Does It Get Any Easier as Children Get Older?

Babies don't stay that way for long. Before you know it, they are toddlers, then they are off to school, and finally they are teenagers with lives of their own. They may need less hands-on care, but children continue to need love, attention, and support until they are adults. Even then they still need good parenting. When you have MS, having a child is a long haul. Don't think just about the birth and the baby, but think ahead to every stage of childhood. Each presents its own challenges. You also have to consider the possibility that your condition will worsen over the years and that the physical side of looking after children will become more and more difficult. Plan ahead for those years, making sure you have practical help for several years down the road.

In some ways, it is easier if the parent has been disabled with MS from the beginning of the child's life. A teenager, to whom outward appearance means so much, can find visible disability in a parent hard to take. Talk to your child. Get your child to express his or her feelings and perceptions. Are they justified?

"The two younger children only remember Tina being in a bad condition. But Tessa, the eldest, remembers when she was taking long walks with her mother. I think that for her it has been very hard to accept the deterioration. She is fifteen and needs to go through that very painful period in her life when she is becoming independent. She sometimes protests violently against her mother. It's hard for her to know how to be aggressive toward such a 'different' mother. Sometimes she can be really nasty."

"I was fine when the baby was born. I could even walk well enough to take him on long walks. But little by little, I noticed I could do less and less. Because I was able to do so much when he was a toddler, he's gotten it into his head that Mom can do anything. Now he looks amazed when I can't do things I used to."

"It got to the point where I just couldn't manage any longer. I was hobbling about like an old lady. My teenage son didn't want to show me in public. He was too embarrassed about the way I looked. So I felt it was better he stayed with his father, who has tons more energy than I do. I left them so that I could lead a slower, quieter life without any domestic hassles. He seems OK."

Telling Your Children You Have MS

Many mothers and fathers get MS when they already have children. The children may remember you as healthy and active and may find it difficult to see you get worse. How you tell your children depends on how old they are and the kind of relationship you have with them. In general, honest, open communication works best.

"We Could All Talk Together about Fear of the Unknowns" ☀ Sue's Story

"I think the biggest plus for me was that I had open communication with both of my kids. Davy was eleven and Steph was eight when I was diagnosed. I can well remember the morning the kids came in to say good-bye on their way to school. It was shortly after my initial problem, and I was still spending a lot of time in bed with extreme weakness in my legs and lack of balance.

"Steph flitted in and got big hugs and kisses and was on her way. Davy hesitated as he sat on the bed and finally blurted out, 'Mommy, are you going to die?' It still takes my breath away. I assured him I was not and told him we would talk when he got home from school. That was OK, because he knew that I was true to my word. They always knew that I would answer any question they had. We could all talk together about fear of the unknowns."

17 ☀ Working for a Living

Women today feel under cultural pressure to "have it all"— a career, marriage, a home, a baby—while staying attractive, fashionable, and sexy. The reality is that many women find juggling all these roles utterly exhausting. If you feel that you must have these things in your life to feel fulfilled, fine. But many mothers with MS take a long, hard look at the reality of their lives and come to the conclusion that trying to do it all is just not possible. Many settle for those things that really matter to them and forget about the rest.

🌾 *"It is rewarding and difficult to juggle it all—motherhood, career, family, friends, spirituality, finances—oh, yeah, and health. The MS just adds one more complicated layer."*

🌾 *"Maybe if I were in a wheelchair I'd be a better mom, because I would be home all the time rather than at work all the time. It has its pros and cons."*

🌾 *"I went back to work as a computer operator when she was six months old. But I had a relapse two weeks afterward. I am now medically retired."*

🌾 *"In order to feel valid, I have to do some work with my brain, contribute socially, and be involved with my children."*

🌾 *"It was such hard work looking after my little boy that when I did go back to work it was like a holiday. Every*

Monday morning I'd go to the office and breathe a sigh of relief that I could take a break."

Many women with MS are working full-time when they get pregnant and have to go back to work six weeks after the baby is born. You may have to reassess this schedule, depending on how you feel. Some mothers find that going out to work and looking after a baby when they come back home is too much. Others find going to work much easier and less exhausting than looking after a baby. Some compromise by working part-time. In time, MS can have a major impact on working life— 75 percent of those affected become too disabled to work.

"I Work Seventy Hours a Week" ✿ Julie's Story

"When Heather was one, I returned to work as a manager at McDonald's. While I was there, I had one episode that started on a very stressful day—my cook didn't show up. I got double vision that lasted for a month. It went away with steroids. Stress has a lot to do with it. My husband is away in Alabama in the military police, and when he's away I have to deal with everything myself—I work 70 hours a week."

Losing the Breadwinner

When the breadwinner has MS, it can cause real hardship if he or she loses a job. It can happen to both men and women.

"The Children Worry about Who Will Provide for Them" ❂ Danny's Story

"I was a trucker in Illinois. At first the MS didn't affect my job at all, but as time went on I became fatigued easily. I told the company I had MS because I had to ask them for special treatment: to work in familiar places where I knew where the restrooms were and to cut back on walking.

"Once employers know you have MS, I think they do everything in their power to get rid of you. They also feel you are an insurance risk and figure that they could hire a healthy guy and not have to deal with special requests. I have lost two jobs because I disclosed I had multiple sclerosis.

"My doctor was hesitant to diagnose me at first because he said it could cause problems with insurance. Insurance companies won't cover you for a preexisting condition. I had good insurance coverage and kept it until I lost my job. I had to buy a wheelchair out of my own pocket because I don't have a job and don't have insurance.

"Our family income has dropped terribly since I lost my job. As a two-salary household, we were earning about $49,000 gross. That dropped to the $17,500 that my wife earns. Owing to the stress of my job loss, I am no longer capable of working and have applied for Social Security Disability. My loss of income has affected the children badly. We have to say no to a lot of things they ask for. We are debating whether we should have a graduation party for them because they are both graduating this June. They worry about whether we will be able to keep our house and whether they will be able to keep going to school with their friends. They worry about who will provide for them now that the company decided I am no longer fit to support my family.

"We have tried to give the children what they want, but we are using credit cards to do it and are putting ourselves in debt trying to give them what they need or want. It makes me feel very sad and bad because I have struggled my whole life to ensure that my children would have a good life. And now, by no choice of my own, I have no control over this. It makes me feel inadequate, depressed, uncertain of my future and my family's future."

Insurance

🖋 *"There's this blackball over your head if you have MS. You can't get health insurance; you can't get life insurance. If you say you have MS, you lose everything. With health insurance, if you say you have MS, the premium goes up. If you don't tell them you have MS they can sue you for nondisclosure."*

Insurance problems can affect not just the person with MS but his or her spouse and children too. An estimated thirty-seven thousand to fifty-two thousand people with MS are uninsured for their health care needs. Even the ones who are insured are underinsured—they are not adequately covered for the costs of long-term health care and support services. The level of disability insurance protection—"income replacement benefits"—is also too low. It replaces only about four dollars of every ten dollars in forgone income. With health insurance reimbursement, people with MS get back less than half their formal costs, leaving the rest—about 57 percent of these MS-related costs—to be paid by the affected person or his or her family. This amounts to about sixteen thousand dollars per person with MS per year. Informal costs, such as help from family, friends, and neighbors, are not reimbursed at all. It makes life a whole lot easier if you can get health insurance before receiving a diagnosis of MS. Some doctors deliberately don't give you a firm diagnosis for this very reason, even when they suspect MS. If you are lucky enough to be in this position, go for the best insurance deal you can get.

🖎 *"When I first got symptoms, it made me and my husband confront the possibility of physical disability. We both took out insurance policies for disability that would have at least provided us enough to live on if one of us became disabled. We did not mention the possibility of MS to the insurance company, although we were truthful about my double vision. We were afraid that our application would be turned down. Insurance companies have the right to turn down applicants if they believe they would be a high risk. But they took me on."*

Most people get health and disability insurance as part of their employment package, but you need to work to get this insurance benefit. In the United States, only about 25 percent of people with MS are employed. This means that 75 to 80 percent are not employed, and are not eligible for company insurance benefits. Full insurance benefits are available only to people who work full-time or almost full-time. Part-time workers are not entitled to the same benefits, which puts additional pressure on women with MS who decide to have children. If they want to work part-time, they lose out—and so do the children.

🖎 *"The financial stressors are the ones that concern me lately in my decision to become a parent. I'm not sure I will always be able to work or raise a child on long-term disability payments—60 percent of my present earnings. I do question whether or not I have the energy to face this challenge."*

Welfare

Going on welfare and getting a disability benefit from Social Security is not always an alternative way of gaining income. Social Security must be convinced that you are unable to do any work.

Finding Time for Yourself

If you are a working mother, you may have very little time left for yourself. When you come home you probably want to spend time with your child and partner, and there are always things in the home that need sorting out. But by the time you've done all that, you'll be lucky if there's any time left for you. If you're not careful, this can affect your health and well-being.

🖋 *"Women tend to relegate themselves behind children and partners, but with MS you have a responsibility not to do that. And it is very, very hard. Between moments of denial, depression, sadness, or the overwhelming task of just trying to fit everything all in, it is easy to neglect your health. I am very bad at this. I need to give myself permission to take care of myself."*

You have a right to free time, but you may need to restructure your life so you get it. Other parents with MS have found the following tips helpful.

- Allow yourself a break. Childcare and chores are never-ending. Unless you call a halt at some time, there will always be something else to do. Giving yourself no time off doesn't make you a better parent.

- Set aside a particular time every day or every week when you have time to yourself.

- Make a regular arrangement with your partner or helper to look after the children and chores during this time.

- Do not ask this as a "favor." Be assertive in your request.

- Other people are more likely to take over if you go out during your time to yourself, for example to go shopping or have your hair done. But you also have to make this arrangement work when you want time alone in your own home.

- During your time to yourself, relax and enjoy what you are doing. Stop clock-watching.

18 ❋ Fathers with MS

The emphasis of this book is on mothers with MS because they are the ones who get pregnant and give birth. Being a father with MS, however, also affects the whole family, in a sometimes more profound way, and is a challenge to all concerned. Wives may have to become their husbands' caregivers and assume the roles of mother, father, housekeeper, breadwinner, and nurse. This puts an extra burden on wives, and a possible strain on relationships, which needs to be talked through before having a baby.

Children are deeply affected by a father's MS too. If he suffers a drop in income, they may have to go without material things that their friends have. Schooling or college education can be hit, and children's lives are changed. On the face of it, this might seem like a change for the worse, but in the long run children in this situation might grow up to have more depth, understanding, and humanity.

It can feel like a blow to a man's pride when his traditional roles are taken from him, and some fathers with MS suffer from feelings of inadequacy because they are not doing what they think they ought to be doing. Thinking like this, however, is counterproductive. Blaming yourself for not being able to play football with your kid will get you nowhere except depressed. You are no less of a loving dad because you cheer from the sidelines. Real parents almost never meet perfectionist standards. You and your kids have to get real. There are many ways to relate to your kids. Love, encouragement, and interest are the most important.

"Now They Feel as Though Their Lives Are Changing for the Worse" ☀ Danny's Story

"The MS does affect me as a dad. I can't play basketball with my son, Richard, or take my daughter, Danielle, to a father/daughter dance. I can't go for walks with them; or if we do go out, someone has to push me in the wheelchair. At first the children were in denial. They wouldn't or couldn't believe it. They wouldn't talk about it and didn't want their friends to know. They understand a little more now, but they are still very scared and worried about their dad and the future.

"My job loss affected my children more than my having MS. As long as I was working, they felt I was doing OK and our lives were going to remain the same. Now they feel as though everything is changing for the worse, and it is causing them grief and worry. They can't have a lot of material things that other kids their age might have because we just don't have the income. And they have lost a lot of my attention because I have been so preoccupied with my job loss, my illness, and the fact that my MS is getting worse.

"The MS has put extra pressure on my wife, Pamela. She was a stay-at-home mom for many years, but she had to go back to school, get some job skills, get a job, and take care of most of the household chores. She has to do the grocery shopping, cleaning, cooking, washing, handling the phone calls, and other business-related tasks. She has to handle what the children need and what I need. She has to deal with my health problems and mood swings. She breaks down and cries a lot and can't believe this is happening.

"It is hard enough trying to be a father and husband and doing what you can to provide and give guidance. I have lived the American dream up until the loss of my job. I worked hard for many years, seven days a week. I have no one other than my wife and children. Yes, there are laws that keep this from happening. But not for the little guy. It's OK to have a health problem as long as you keep it to yourself."

"My Daughter Took My Illness Very Badly"
☀ Dave's Story

"One night I went to bed, and when I woke up the next morning I couldn't feel a thing along the whole of my left side. My daughter took my illness very badly. We used to do a lot of sports together—playing squash and running—and she could see all this being taken from her.

"My MS has caused a lot of extra strain on my wife, and I'm not happy about that. She has to do everything and has had to take on my role, doing the things that I used to do, like the driving, gardening, mowing the lawn. It is a blow to my pride because I'm an old-fashioned type who likes to support his wife and family and do all the manly things. I try to do a bit of do-it-yourself around the house, but it's not so easy now.

"We deliberately never asked for the children to help because we think they should lead normal lives and not take on the burden of me. They shouldn't push a wheelchair—it won't do their backs any good. But the children are certainly more aware of disability, and the older one is thinking of taking up a career in occupational therapy. What happened to me has had a huge effect on shaping what she wanted to do with her life."

"This Has Been Harder Than Marine Corps Boot Camp" ☀ Rocky's Story

"My wife and neurologist won't let me work full-time anymore —the wimps! They're afraid I'll get worse because they feel I'm working too hard now. (How could it get worse!) I work as an auto mechanic and have gone from working ten hours a day to six hours a day. Because I'm working part-time now, it has affected my income. It's hard to pay *all* the bills. Some don't get paid.

"So many symptoms all happening at once have made me very depressed at times, which makes me not want to do anything. But I have tried not to let it keep me down! I still do all the things I like to do, like hunting, and I still work as hard as I can. All I can say is that this has been the hardest thing I have ever had to go through, even harder than Marine Corps boot camp. And my three wonderful children seem so sad. It is hard to show them that I will be OK."

19 ✺ Being a Parent with MS

This last chapter provides a final positive note. Although having MS can be difficult, it is still possible to lead a happy and fulfilling life. Many of the people interviewed for this book testify to that.

🏵 *"I don't know how to be a mother without having MS."*

🏵 *"When you're a mother with MS, your children can be nicer kids. They are more aware of other people's problems, more compassionate and humane."*

🏵 *"People see a wheelchair careening along with a boy on the back and a little girl on my lap. It breaks the stereotype. They say, 'Hang on a minute.'"*

🏵 *"My daughter is so caring. She is really sensitive to my needs."*

🏵 *"In many ways it's been good for the children that my wife, Tina, has MS. They don't stare at disabled people when they see them in the street. Our children have also met and gotten to know many MSers and they have seen that this illness is very different from case to case."*

Are Children Better for Having a Parent with MS?

Although there are undoubted practical difficulties to being a parent with MS, it is also possible to look at it another way, to see the advantages. Many parents comment that their children have a more open and healthy attitude toward disabled people because of their own experience.

🖋 *"For Craig, a wheelchair is part of the furniture. He sees it as part of normal life. He doesn't stare at people in wheelchairs. He is a very caring child. He'll say things like 'Can you play this game with me, Mom, as long as your legs aren't hurting?' And even though he's only three, he always says 'Can I help you, Mom?' We just love our little boy so much."*

🖋 *"My eldest son was nine and a half when he had to do a presentation at school on the person he most admired. He came home from school and said, 'Mom, I did you. Because you try so hard, and you do as much as you can.' The teacher said it was lovely."*

🖋 *"You do need to ask other people for help, and I've enjoyed that aspect of MS. My daughter said, 'We meet so many people!' I'm always asking people for help, for example, if I need help getting the wheelchair out of the car. I'll ask anyone who just happens to be passing. This has lots of advantages. I'm glad my daughter can assess what kind of people will help."*

Parenthood—A Positive Experience

Ironic though it may sound, women with MS can be better parents than others. They have time for their children and perhaps savor the joys of parenthood more acutely. Without a doubt, countless men and women with MS find parenthood a positive experience—regardless of their disability.

"My Children Have Grown Up without Questioning My Disability" ✿ Eleanor's Story

"As someone with MS, my experiences of being pregnant can only be described as good. Following the birth, my MS symptoms returned. Pushing a pram or stroller helped me to walk. And later, when the children held my hand, they unwittingly helped me keep my balance. My children have grown up without questioning my disability. Now that they are older, they understand me quite well and can often supply my needs without my having to ask."

In a report on a conference about disabled people, pregnancy, and early parenthood that took place in 1993 Elizabeth Brice, a mother with MS and a freelance journalist, says

Many households with a disabled parent are very open, with people constantly coming around to give help or support, and this must be better for a child than a claustrophobic and inward-looking environment. There are advantages to being a disabled parent when the children are older too. Disabled people are more ready to confront and deal with problems, because they've had to deal with problems themselves, and so would be more likely to be able to tackle any problems their children have, which 'normal, well-adjusted' families might sweep under the carpet.

"I had the last baby when I was forty—nine years after number three. It was the best thing that could have happened to me. So I say, 'Go ahead and enjoy the delights of a family while you can.'"

🖋 *"So many people rush around dragging small children in tow, but disabled people tend to move at a slower pace, much more like that of their children, and they probably have more time to spend with them. All children are precious to their parents, but if you've had to fight against the odds to have your children, they're bound to be somehow especially precious.*

"We Try to Protect Every Ounce of Quality Time" ☼ Sue's Story

"My daughter, Steph, and I have been very good friends as she has gotten older. She likes shopping with me because it is real one-on-one time. We find the chairs so I can sit, and she brings choices to me. Then we move to the next store at the mall and do the same thing. Sometimes I sit and watch people while she shops. But we still get our lattes (after all, we do live in Seattle—the latte capital of the world!) and 'do lunch.' Is it the same as it would be if I could be on my feet and navigate the stores all afternoon or all day? Of course not, but we try to protect every ounce of quality time together."

Get On with Your Life

The people who seem to do best with MS are the ones who get on with their lives. They accept their limitations and do what they can. Those who seem to have the hardest time whine and bemoan their lot. They see the negative in everything and think only of all the things they can't do. Try to keep MS in perspective. It is not your whole life, and it need not dominate everything you think and do. Decide to make the most of life and don't let MS stop you from living the life you want. For some, this attitude will encompass having a child. For others, it will not. Do what you want to do, no matter what other people may think. Listen to your doctor and discuss things with your family and others with whom you are close. Remember that no one else can make decisions for you.

It's your life. Live it.

❋ Appendix A: Multiple Sclerosis Organizations and Information Services

Organizations

The National Multiple Sclerosis Society
Funds research and provides information and resources. The Society has 140 local chapters and branches throughout the United States.
733 3rd Avenue, New York, NY 10017
Tel: 800-Fight MS (800-344-4867)
E-mail: info@nmss.org
Website: www.nmss.org

Multiple Sclerosis Association of America
Offers peer counseling, a buddy system, equipment, support groups, etc. More alternative-oriented than the MS Society.
National Headquarters: 706 Haddonfield Road, Cherry Hill, NJ 08002
Tel: 800-LEARN MS (800-833-4672) or 609-488-4500;
Fax: 609-661-9797
Website: www.msaa@msaa.com

Multiple Sclerosis Foundation Inc.
Provides information and support.
6350 N. Andrews Avenue, Fort Lauderdale, FL 33309
Tel: 954-776-6805 or 800-441-7055
E-mail: msfact@icanect.net
Website: www.msfacts.org

International MS Support Foundation
Publishes *Multiple Sclerosis News from Arizona.*
PO Box 90154, Tucson, AZ 85752-0154
Website: www.msnews.org

Multiple Sclerosis Association of King County
Has support groups, educational workshops, and therapy for people with MS and their families.
753 North 35, Suite 208, Seattle, WA 98103-8802

Tel: 206-633-2606; fax: 206-633-2929
Website: www.msa-sea.org

Eastern Paralyzed Veterans Association
Publishes *MS Quarterly Report.*
65-20 Astoria Boulevard, Jackson Heights, NY 11370-1177
Tel: 718-803-3782; fax: 718-803-0414
Website: www.epva.org/msarticle.html

National Rehabilitation Information Center
8455 Colesville Road, Suite 935, Silver Spring, MD 20910-3319
Tel: 800-346-2742 or 301-588-9284; fax: 301-587-1967
Website: www.naric.com/naric

ABLEDATA Adaptive Equipment Center
Newington Children's Hospital
181 E. Cedar Street, Newington, CT 06111
Tel: 800-344-5404, 860-667-5405 in Connecticut
Website: www.abledata.com
ABLEDATA is a database with information on fifteen thousand
disability products.

American Holistic Medical Association
4101 Lake Boone Trail, Suite 201, Raleigh, NC 27607
Tel: 919-787-5181

Foundation for Toxic-free Dentistry
PO Box 608010, Orlando, FL 32860-8010
Tel: 407-299-4149

Clinics and Research Centers

Swank Multiple Sclerosis Clinic
Treats MS with low-fat diet and plasma. Publishes excellent
newsletter with advice on management of MS and hints on
daily living.
13655 SW Jenkins Road, Beaverton, OR 97005
Tel: 503-520-1050; fax: 503-520-1223

Center for Neurologic Study (CNS)
Provides information and support services for people in South-
ern California.
11211 Sorrento Valley Rd., Suite H, San Diego, CA 92121
Tel: 619-455-5463; fax: 619-455-1713
Website: www.cnsonline.org

Rocky Mountain MS Center
Comprehensive center dedicated to the study and treatment of
MS. Provides patient care and support services.
701 East Hampden Avenue, Suite 430, Englewood,
CO 80110-2790
Tel: 303-788-4030

Consortium of Multiple Sclerosis Centers
Provides networking for all health care professionals specializ-
ing in the care of MS patients.
Multiple Sclerosis Comprehensive Care Center, Holy Name
Hospital, 718 Teaneck Road, Teaneck, NJ 07666
Tel: 201-837-0727; fax: 201-837-8504
E-mail: halper@holyname.org

Websites

Computer Literate Advocates for Multiple Sclerosis (CLAMS)
Lists all sources of information about MS on the Web. Runs
the MS Web Ring. The best route to all information about MS
on the Internet.
www.clams.org

MS Crossroads
Essential links and archive data about MS on the Web. Run by
Aapo Halko, a Finnish man with MS.
www.helsinki.fi/~ahalko/ms.html

MS Direct
Helps people find their way around information about MS on
the Internet.
www.aquila.com/dean.sporleder/ms-home/

Colorado HealthNet News
Has Q&A on MS.
www.coloradohealthnet.org

The MSers Chat Room
www.geocities.com~klinks.html/msed.html

The "Red Boa" Society—MS support group
www.shore.net/~robertj/boapage.html

MedSupport Friends Supporting Friends (FSF) International
www.medsupport.org/forums.htm
24-hour MS Support Hotline: 800-793-0766

International Federation of Multiple Sclerosis Societies
Has thirty-six member societies around the world.
www.infosci.org/MS-internat/FAQ-1.2.html

The Good Docs List
Lists good doctors for MS state by state.
www.clams.org/goodocs.html

Noreen's Home on the Net
Excellent list of information on MS from the Internet compiled
by Noreen Fogeson.
www.crl.com/~rbarnes/noreen.html

☀ Appendix B: Useful Books and Publications

Books

The National Multiple Sclerosis Society has several books and leaflets relevant to parenthood and MS. For a full list of their publications, ask for their "Information In Print" leaflet from the National MS Society head office.
Customer Service Inquiries: 212-986-3240

Multiple Sclerosis: A Guide for Families
Edited by Rosalind C. Kalb, Ph.D.
New York: Demos Vermande, 1998.
A truly excellent book, covering every aspect of having MS and its impact on the family. Essential reading.

Multiple Sclerosis: The Questions You Have—The Answers You Need
By Rosalind C. Kalb, Ph.D.
New York: Demos Vermande, 1996.

Mother to Be: A Guide to Pregnancy and Birth for Women with Disabilities
By Judith Rogers and Molleen Matsumura
New York: Demos Vermande, 1991.

Multiple Sclerosis: The Self Help Guide to Its Management
By Judy Graham
Rochester, Vt.: Healing Arts Press, 1989.

The New Road To Wellness
By Roy L. Swank and Barbara Brewer Dugan
New York: Doubleday, 1998.

Sick and Tired of Feeling Sick and Tired: Living with Invisible Chronic Illness
By Paul J. Donoghue and Mary E. Siegel (who has MS)
New York: Norton, 1992.
Written by two psychologists, it looks at the dilemmas facing those with an invisible chronic illness.

Sexuality and Multiple Sclerosis, 3rd ed.
By M. Barrett
Toronto: Multiple Sclerosis Society of Canada, 1991.
Available from: 250 Bloor Street East, Suite 1000, Toronto,
Ontario, M4W 3P9, Canada
Tel: 416-922-6065

*Living Well with MS: A Guide for Patient, Caregiver and
Family*
By David L. Carroll, Jon Dorman, and M. D. Dorman
New York: HarperCollins, 1993.

*Health Insurance: How to Get It, Keep It, or Improve What
You've Got*
By Robert Enteen, Ph.D.
New York: Demos Vermande, 1996.

Newsletters

The Swank MS Clinic Newsletter
13655 SW Jenkins Road, Beaverton, OR 97005
From the professor who champions the low-fat diet, lots of
everyday hints on how to manage MS.

MS'ers Newsletter
Published by John Pageler. Full of tips from people who follow
John's program of milk- and dairy-free diet, vitamin supplements, stress management, massage, and other complementary therapies.
6200 102 Terrace N., Pinellas Park, FL 33782
Tel: 813-546-0994

MS One To One
Newsletter from: 1635 South Bertelsen Road
Eugene, OR 97402-2821
E-mail: MSOneToOne@aol.com
Website: www.msonetoone/index.htm

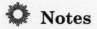 **Notes**

Chapter 1

1. J. Whitaker, "Effects of Pregnancy and Delivery on Disease Activity in Multiple Sclerosis," *New Engl J Med* 339, no. 5 (1998): 339–40.
2. M. A. A. Walverdeen et al., "Magnetic Resonance Evaluation of Disease Activity During Pregnancy in Multiple Sclerosis," *Neurology* 44 (1994): 327–29.
3. K. Birk and R. Rudick, "Pregnancy and Multiple Sclerosis" [review], *Arch Neurol* 43 (1986): 719–26.
4. P. Duquette and M. Girard, "Hormonal Factors in Susceptibility to Multiple Sclerosis," *Curr Opin Neurol Neurosurg* 6 (1993): 195–201.
5. K. Birk et al., "The Clinical Course of Multiple Sclerosis During Pregnancy and the Puerperium," *Arch Neurol* 47 (1990): 738–42.
6. E. Roullet et al., "Pregnancy and Multiple Sclerosis: A Longitudinal Study of 125 Remittent Patients," *J Neurol Neurosurg Psychiatry* 56 (1993): 1062–65.
7. R. Rudick, "Pregnancy and Multiple Sclerosis" [letter], *Arch Neurol* 52 (1995): 849–50.
8. S. Bernardi et al., "The Influence of Pregnancy on Relapse in Multiple Sclerosis: A Cohort Study," *Acta Neurol Scand* 84 (1991): 403–6.
9. Whitaker, 339–40.
10. Roullet et al., 1062–65.
11. Whitaker, 339–40.
12. Roullet et al., 1062–65.
13. Birk et al., "The Clinical Course of Multiple Sclerosis During Pregnancy and the Puerperium," 738–42.
14. Birk and Rudick, 719–26.
15. Roullet et al., 1062–65.
16. L. Nelson, G. Franklin, and M. Jones, "Risk of Multiple Sclerosis Exacerbation During Pregnancy and Breastfeeding," *JAMA* 259, no. 23 (1988): 3441–43.
17. Birk et al., "The Clinical Course of Multiple Sclerosis During Pregnancy and the Puerperium," 738–42.
18. Birk and Rudick, 719–26.

19. Ibid.
20. Nelson, Franklin, and Jones, 3441–43.
21. Whitaker, 339–40.
22. E. Stenager, E. N. Stenager, and K. Jensen, "Effect of Pregnancy on the Prognosis for Multiple Sclerosis: A 5 Year Follow-Up Investigation," *Acta Neurol Scand* 90 (1994): 305–8.
23. J. Worthington et al., "Pregnancy and Multiple Sclerosis: A 3 Year Prospective Study," *J Neurol* 241 (1994): 228–33.
24. E. Stenager, E. N. Stenager, and K. Jensen, "Pregnancy, birth, gynecologic operations and multiple sclerosis" [letter], *Acta Obstet Gynecol Scand* 71 (1992): 88–89.
25. S. Poser and W. Poser, "Multiple Sclerosis and Gestation," *Neurology* 33 (1983): 1422–27.
26. B. Runmarker and O. Andersen, "Pregnancy Is Associated with a Lower Risk of Onset and a Better Prognosis in Multiple Sclerosis," *Brain* 118 (1995): 253–61.
27. Roullet et al., 1062–65.
28. Runmarker and Andersen, "Pregnancy Is Associated with a Lower Risk of Onset and a Better Prognosis in Multiple Sclerosis," 253–61.
29. P. Verdru et al., "Pregnancy and Multiple Sclerosis: The Influence on Long Term Disability," *Clin Neurol Neurosurg* 96 (1994): 38–41.
30. Poser and Poser, 33: 1422–27.
31. D. S. Thompson et al., "The Effects of Pregnancy in Multiple Sclerosis: A Retrospective Study," *Neurology* 36 (1986): 1097–99.
32. Poser and Poser, 1422–27.
33. Runmarker and Andersen, "Prognosis Factors in a Multiple Sclerosis Incidence Cohort with Twenty-five Years' Follow-up," *Brain* 116 (1993): 117–34.

Chapter 2

1. A. Sadovnick et al., "Pregnancy and Multiple Sclerosis: A Prospective Study," *Arch Neurol* 51 (1994): 1120–24.
2. A. Sadovnick and P. Baird, "The Familial Nature of Multiple Sclerosis: Age-corrected Empiric Recurrence Risks for Children and Siblings of Patients," *Neurology* (1988): 990–91.

Chapter 3

1. K. Birk, R. N. Smeltzer, and R. Rudick, "Pregnancy and Multiple Sclerosis," *Semin Neurol* 8, no. 3 (1988): 205–13.
2. Birk and Rudick, 719–26.
3. Meg Goodman, *Mothers' Pride and Others' Prejudice: A Survey of Disabled Mothers' Experiences of Maternity* (London, UK: Disability Working Group of the Disability Alliance, 1997).
4. Roullet et al., 1062–65.
5. Birk and Rudick, 719–26.
6. Birk, Smeltzer, and Rudick, 205–13.

Chapter 4

1. Roy S. Swank and Barbara B. Dugan. *The Multiple Sclerosis Diet Book—A Low-Fat Diet for the Treatment of Multiple Sclerosis* (New York: Doubleday, 1989).
2. R. Swank and B. Dugan, "Effect of Low Saturated Fat Diet in Early and Late Cases of Multiple Sclerosis," *Lancet* 336 (1990): 37–39.
3. *The Swank MS Clinic Newsletter,* spring 1998. The Swank M.S. Foundation, 13655 SW Jenkins Road, Beaverton, OR 97005.
4. Melvyn R. Werbach, M.D., *Nutritional Influences on Illness* (New Canaan, Conn.: Keats Publishing, 1987).
5. M. Esparza et al., "Nutrition, Latitude and Multiple Sclerosis Mortality: An Ecologic Study," *Am J Epidemiol* 142 (1995): 733–37.
6. R. Gonsette and P. Delmotte, "Recent Advances in Multiple Sclerosis Therapy," in *Excerpta Medica* (UK: Elsevier Science Publishers, 1989), 365–66.
7. R. Jones et al., "Blood Studies in Multiple Sclerosis—The Present Status," in *Current Concepts in Multiple Sclerosis,* H. Wietholter et al., eds. (UK: Elsevier Science Publishers, 1991), 103–5.
8. M. Enig, "Fatty Acid Composition of Selected Food Items with Emphasis on Trans Octadecenoate and Trans Octadecedienoate," unpublished doctoral thesis, University of Maryland, 1981.

9. Leon Chaitow, *Candida Albicans: Could Yeast Be Your Problem?* (Rochester, Vt.: Healing Arts Press, 1998), 2.

10. D. Eisenberg et al., "Trends in Alternative Medicine Use in the United States, 1990–1997," *J Am Med Assoc* 280 (1998): 1569–75.

11. R. E. Miller, "An Investigation into the Management of the Spasticity Experienced by some Patients with Multiple Sclerosis Using Acupuncture Based on Traditional Chinese Medicine," *Comp Ther Med* 4, no. 1 (1996): 58–62.

12. F. Lublin, "Preliminary Test Results of Bee Venom in Mice with MS-Like Disease," *Neurology* 50 (1998): A424.

13. U. Jobst, "Posturographic Biofeedback Training in Equilibrium Disorders," *Fortschritte der Neurologie-Psychiatrie* 57, no. 2 (1989): 74–80.

14. J. T. Ungerleider et al., "Delta-9-THC in the Treatment of Spasticity Associated with Multiple Sclerosis," *Advances In Alcohol & Substance Abuse* 7, no. 1 (1987): 39–50.

15. R. Brenneisen et al., "The Effect of Orally and Rectally Administered Delta-9-Tetrahydrocannabinol on Spasticity: A Pilot Study with 2 Patients," *Int J Clin Pharmacol Ther* 34, no. 10 (1996): 446–50.

16. D. Bates et al., "A Double-Blind Controlled Trial of Long Chain n-3 Polyunsaturated Fatty Acids in the Treatment of Multiple Sclerosis," *J Neuro Neurosurg Psychiatry* 52, no. 1 (1989): 18–22.

17. D. Bates et al., "Polyunsaturated Fatty Acids In Treatment of Acute Remitting Multiple Sclerosis," *Brit Med J* 2, no. 6149 (1978): 1390–91.

18. R. H. Dworkin et al., "Linoleic Acid and Multiple Sclerosis: A Reanalysis of Three Double-Blind Trials," *Neurology* 34, no. 11 (1984): 1441–45.

19. D. Horrobin, "Multiple Sclerosis: The Rational Basis for Treatment with Colchicine and Evening Primrose Oil," *Medical Hypotheses* 5 (1979): 365–78.

20. A. Alquist and G. Kraft, "Exercise Study," paper available from Multiple Sclerosis Association of King County, 753 North 35th, Suite 208, Seattle, WA 98103-8802.

21. A. Saine, "Homoeopathic Treatment of the Multiple Sclerosis Patient," *Homoeopath* 10, no. 1 (1990): 20–21.

22. L. Johnston, "Conium in a Case of Multiple Sclerosis," *J Am Institute Homeopathy* 83, no. 1 (1990): 12–15.

23. J. P. Boissel et al., "Overview of Data from Homoeopathic

Medicine Trials: Reports on the Efficacy of Homoeopathic Interventions Over No Treatment of Placebo," Report of the Homoeopathic Medicine Research Group, European Commission, Brussels, 1996.

24. T. L. Richards et al., "Double-Blind Study of Pulsing Magnetic Field Effects on Multiple Sclerosis," *J Alt Comp Med* 3, no. 1 (1997): 21–29.

25. M. Hernandez-Reif et al., "Multiple Sclerosis Patients Benefit From Massage Therapy," *J Bodywork Movement Ther* 2, no. 3 (1998): 168–74.

26. A. Vickers, *Massage and Aromatherapy: A Guide for Health Professionals* (London: Chapman and Hall, 1996).

27. B. Brouwer and V. Sousa de Andrade, "The Effects of Slow Stroking on Spasticity in Patients with Multiple Sclerosis: A Pilot Study," *Physiother Theory Pract* 11, no. 13 (1995): 13–21.

28. J. Crawford and G. McIvor, "Group Psychotherapy: Benefits in Multiple Sclerosis," *Arch Phys Med Rehab* 66, no. 12 (1985): 98810–13.

29. I. Siev-Ner et al., "Reflexology Treatment Relieves Symptoms of Multiple Sclerosis: A Randomized Controlled Study" (presented at the 4th Annual Symposium on Complementary Healthcare, 10–12 December 1997, Exeter, UK) *Focus Alt Compl Ther* 2, no. 4 (1997): 196.

30. B. Maguire, "The Effects of Imagery on Attitudes and Moods in Multiple Sclerosis," *Alt Ther Health Med* 2, no. 5 (1996): 75–79.

31. D. E. Moulin et al., "Pain Syndromes in Multiple Sclerosis," *Neurology* 38 (1988): 1830–34.

32. P. G. Mattison, "TENS in the Management of Painful Muscle Spasm in Patients with MS," *Clin Rehab* 7 (1993): 45–48.

Chapter 5

1. Poser and Poser, 1422–47.

Chapter 6

1. Birk and Rudick, 719–26.

2. Birk et al., "Pregnancy and Multiple Sclerosis," *Semin Neurol* 8, no. 3 (1988): 205–13.
3. M. Crawford et al., "Essential Fatty Acids in Early Development," in *Polyunsaturated Fatty Acids In Human Nutrition,* U. Bracco and R. J. Deckelbaum, eds. (New York: Vevey/Raven Press, 1992).
4. M. Crawford et al., "N-6 and N-3 Fatty Acids During Early Human Development," *J Int Med* 225, Suppl. 1 (1989): 159–60.

Chapter 7

1. Berlex website: www.berlex.com
2. Biogen website: www.biogen.com
3. Copaxone website: www.tevapharmusa.com/copaxone
4. Poser and Poser, 1422–27.
5. "Antineoplastic and Immunosuppressive Agents: Azathioprine," *IARC Monographs* 26 (1981): 47–78.
6. Duquette and Girard, 195–201.
7. L. Grush et al., "St. John's Wort During Pregnancy," *JAMA* 280 (1998): 1566.
8. M. Cirigliano and A. Sun, "Advising Patients about Herbal Therapies" [letter], *JAMA* 280 (1998): 1565–66.

Chapter 8

1. Birk and Rudick, 719–26.
2. S. Cook et al., "Multiple Sclerosis and Pregnancy," chapter 8 in *Neurological Complications of Pregnancy,* O. Devinsky, E. Feldmann, and B. Hainline, eds. (New York: Raven Press, 1994), 83–95.
3. Birk et al., "Pregnancy and Multiple Sclerosis," 205–13.
4. Ibid.
5. M. Marks et al., "Women Whose Mental Illnesses Recur After Childbirth and Partners' Levels of Expressed Emotion During Late Pregnancy," *Brit J Psychiatry,* 161 (1992): 211–16.
6. Cook et al., 83–95.

Chapter 9

1. A. Pisacane et al., "Breast-Feeding and Multiple Sclerosis," *Brit Med J* 308 (1994): 1411–12.
2. Nelson, Franklin, and Jones, 3441–43.
3. Berlex website: www.berlex.com
4. Biogen website: www.biogen.com
5. Copaxone website: www.tevapharmusa.com/copaxone

Chapter 11

1. L. Grush et al., "St. John's Wort During Pregnancy" [letter], *JAMA,* 280 (1998): 1566.

Chapter 12

1. B. Weinshenker et al., "The Influence of Pregnancy on Disability from Multiple Sclerosis: A Population-Based Study in Middlesex County, Ontario," *Neurology* 39 (1989): 1438–40.
2. Thompson et al., 1097–99.
3. Goodman, *Mothers' Pride and Others' Prejudice: A Survey of Disabled Mothers' Experiences of Maternity.*
4. Ibid.
5. Poser and Poser, 1422–27.

✺ Index